Sharing MS

Sharing MS

Three women share their conversations
of living with
Multiple Sclerosis

by

Linda Ironside

with

Flora McLeod and Julie Zuby

The SECOND in the series:
White Knight's Remarkable Women

White Knight Publications
2004, Toronto, Canada

Published in 2004 by White Knight Publications,
a division of Bill Belfontaine Ltd.
Suite 103, One Benvenuto Place
Toronto Ontario Canada M4V 2L1
T. 416-925-6458 F. 416-925-4165 E-mail: whitekn@istar.ca

Ordering information
Hushion House
c/o Georgetown Terminal Warehouses
34 Armstrong Avenue, Georgetown ON, L7G 4R9
T. 866-485-5556 F. 866-485-6665
E-mail: orders@gtwcanada.com

National Library of Canada Cataloguing in Publication

Ironside, Linda L.
Sharing MS : three women share their stories
about multiple sclerosis / Linda Ironside.

(White Knight's remarkable women ; 1)
ISBN 0-9730949-7-4

1. Multiple sclerosis—Patients—Biography. I. Title. II. Series.

RC377.I76 2003   362.1'96834'00922   C2003-901993-4

———————————————

COVER AND INTERIOR DESIGN
Karen Petherick, Intuitive Design International Ltd.

TEXT FONTS
Transit 521

COVER PHOTOGRAPH
2004 © Getty Images

EDITING
Bill Belfontaine

PRINTED AND BOUND IN CANADA

Dedicated to the memory of my father,
Robert Watkinson, 1914-1979

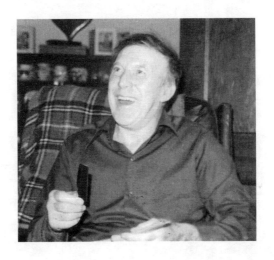

CONTENTS

ACKNOWLEDGEMENTS

First, of course, I thank Julie Zuby and Flora McLeod who were willing to share their experience with me through e-mail. They went further and agreed to let our private correspondence become public; they have always been patient and obliging with my requests.

My undying gratitude to Tanis Ironside for her ongoing support, and more specifically, for her vital introduction to White Knight Publishing.

Michael Kaufman-Lacusta is the Vancouver editor who took on the very difficult job of selecting e-mail letters to form coherent sections, and then showing me where and how to link them all together. I thank him for his insight and for sticking with the project.

Dr. Ma of Dr. Yan Bin Ma Natural Therapy Centre has given me acupuncture treatments and herbal remedies, which ensured I had the energy to complete the writing and fulfill publishing needs. Hers has been a vital, though indirect, contribution.

Andrew Allan was my computer guru, who saved the book from both virus attack and my ineptitude.

Janene Spring-Welbedagt, RN (former Manager of Individual and Family Services, MS Society of Canada, BC Division) gave me valuable feedback in the early, formative stages of the book.

A big thank you goes to Bill Belfontaine of White Knight Publications for taking on this project, for being MS-sensitive in his potentially stressful requests, and for helping with the finishing touches. Also to members of his White Knight team: Karen Petherick, of Intuitive Design, who made the book visually appealing, and Darlene Montgomery, the publicist, who ensured it would reach readers.

FOREWORD

What This Book Is About

The book is intended for anyone who wants to know what living with MS is like. Although my collaborators in Part Two and I are women, there is little that we talk about does not apply equally to men with MS. It can also be of benefit to a person who does not have the disease themselves but is related to or is a friend of someone who does, and for anyone who wants to learn more about what it's really like to live with the disease; it will give the disease a human face to professionals who are seeking more insight. For people directly and indirectly affected by MS, this book will be a source of ideas and questions – medical, social, family and job related. Those who have lived with MS will recognize themselves and perhaps gain another perspective on their lives. More generally, the book is for anyone who finds the human experience interesting – in this case, that of coping with disability and disease – coping and prevailing!

The book is divided into two parts: "Reflections", and "MS Chat". The former is a collection of my own thoughts and observations, including a lengthy description of my diagnosis, which is noteworthy because it happened in China. Part Two is taken from my e-mail correspondence with two other women who have MS, Flora McLeod MSW of Vancouver and Julie Zuby BSc., who lives in Michigan. These chats have been edited to put together what we have had to say on many pertinent subjects – drugs, diet, mobility aids, bladder, etc. You will find the common approach running through both parts is our upbeat attitude, the "coping and prevailing" I mentioned above. You will see in Part Two comments which will remind you of those made in Part One, but now in a less philosophical, more daily living context.

A word of warning: Part Two is not for the faint of heart. We do speak candidly about bodily functions and the impact of MS. It may also prove difficult for those who are not (yet) able to laugh at the many indignities that the disease thrusts on us and the foibles that it inevitably uncovers. All three of us have had MS for a number of years and, for the most part, have come to terms with the vagaries of the disease. But someone who is newly diagnosed may be shocked by details on things they have never heard of and may well never have to deal with. I suggest moving on to an easier topic.

The title, "Sharing MS" refers to the sharing I have done with Flora and Julie and that which all three of us are doing with you, the reader. Small scale and large scale sharing. Much Sharing you might call it.

Linda Ironside <linside@uniserve.com>

MS 101

A few words about the disease for those who need an introduction to what we'll be talking about. If you want a detailed account of current theories of the cause of MS and the chemistry behind the treatments, this is not the book to help you. (I'm an expert in the practice of MS, not the theory. Flora, Julie and I share our coping strategies and observations on life with MS; they know better than to try to teach me, a language teacher, the science behind it.) You probably already know that MS is a chronic inflammatory disease. It's the most common disease of the central nervous system striking people most often between the ages of twenty-five and forty-five, and is more common in women than men.

Briefly, the disease affects the myelin sheath, the protection around the nerve fibres. In places the myelin breaks down, which slows the nerve impulses. When I have trouble walking it is mostly because the nerve signals which activate the muscles are having trouble getting through. Different people have trouble in different parts of the body, because different nerves are affected. Additionally, the same person may have trouble in different parts of the body at different times. It's a capricious disease: one person has vision problems, another has reduced mobility. One may have no overt symptoms at all many years after diagnosis, and another may progressively lose control in various parts of the body from the onset of the disease.

Some interesting facts about MS:

- ❑ Multiple Sclerosis (MS) means many scars.
- ❑ The disease is much more common in women than in men.
- ❑ MS affects over 50,000 Canadians, 350,000 Americans.
- ❑ The further the geographic area is from the equator, the more cases of MS per capita.
- ❑ Common symptoms include muscle weakness; fatigue; numbness; loss of balance; problems with vision, speech, bowel, or bladder.
- ❑ Statistics show that two-thirds (or so) of individuals with MS are ambulatory 20 years after their diagnosis.
- ❑ People often experience a worsening of symptoms when hot.
- ❑ MS is not inherited, though there are many families with more than one member who has the disease. Research has not yet determined the genetic link; it seems to be some kind of predisposition to the disease.

A Few Words about me:

I was diagnosed in 1980, at the age of 33, in China, where I was teaching English at Zhongshan (Sun Yat-Sen) University in Guangzhou (Canton). My MS journey started, then, as a fascinating adventure. MS brought real changes in my life only in 1987, when I suffered several attacks in Vancouver, where I was living and teaching. My lowest point was the six months I spent in a group home, depressed, afraid, and confused about what was happening and what options I had. Life is so very much better now! I have used a cane, a walker, and scooter for extended travel since my troubles in 1987. I still drive and take along the cane, walker or scooter to use at my destination.

I went on Long Term Disability in 1995, ending a career of twenty-six years in education, lastly as a college instructor of English as a Second Language. I am divorced and have no children. I live with my dog in an adapted apartment, which came in very handy during an attack in 1988, when I depended on a wheelchair to get around. Twice a week I have a homemaker to look after my cleaning, laundry, and odd jobs, like watering the plants. A pleasant assistant, she saves me valuable, limited energy, and is essential in assuring me quality of life.

Like Flora, I am a Canadian, and live on the Canada Pension Plan (CPP) and Long Term Disability (LTD).

Sharing
MS

PART ONE ~ REFLECTIONS

I REMEMBER A PLAY

Even after more than 12 years of being visibly disabled, I still occasionally have an out-of-body experience, where I look at myself from somewhere out there and am amazed to see who I have become. It still does not seem real to me, this person having trouble getting out of the car with dog in tow, trouble getting to the phone in four rings, trouble climbing stairs. Is this denial or just a melodramatic personality? Twelve years is just not long enough to fully accept the 'new' me.

As I reflect back on my life prior to diagnosis, I am often struck by memories of early contact, albeit ignorant, with disability. Like the high school play that became such an ironic precursor.

grew up in Stratford, Ontario, home of the world-famous Shakespeare Theatre. Grade 9 was my first chance to walk the boards. I played Ethel in a play called "The Window", thrilled with both the teacher-director and student male lead, a sophisticated older man to a naïve Grade 9'er. Ethel was in a wheelchair for the whole play. Hard to remember what that meant to me at that time – I think it was mainly a prop, a sort of toy. I'm sure I had no sense of what it might mean, what it might feel like to have to get around full-time in one. I'd never known anyone who used one; they were the stuff of movies . . . and plays.

What is interesting and ironic to me now about that particular play is that it turned out that Ethel was not really a paraplegic; at the end of the play, in a moment of high drama hardly matched by the thespians down by the river, she stands up, unassisted. Her faked disability had something to do with her alibi for a most heinous crime, which escapes me now.

That's how I feel now when I look down on myself – like a fake, who doesn't really need to use a scooter, or a walker. That at the deepest level of meaning, I am just using disability as a disguise, for the attention and perks (handicapped parking, income tax discount, etc.) it brings.

I first used a wheelchair without a script in August of 1988, during a relapse of MS. It was decidedly less fun than the rehearsals (during which other cast members and I had a great time doing wheelies and trying to lay rubber on those long, shiny, school corridors). I found that not only could I not do wheelies, I was continually forgetting to keep my feet on the rest, and was running over one or the other of them in my attempt to turn or back up. (It made me wonder where Ethel had learned to drive well enough to be so convincing.)

"The Window" was my first play and I knew little more about acting than that there were lines to memorize and make-up to put on. The present situation has me feeling no less the amateur, even after years with the scooter. It's been like opening night without the rehearsals! I was cast for this play more than twenty years ago, but given no script. What's worse, there is no director! It's been straight improvisation all the way – for me, for my friends (who have supporting roles) and, unfortunately, for the doctors. We are all "actors in search of a script."

Linda L. Ironside

And I just can't shake the feeling that I could take off the make-up and step out of this role if I just waited long enough.

MODELS FROM MY PAST

When I reflect on my past, I also remember real people in my life long before I was diagnosed with MS who were early connections with disability. At the time I may have taken little notice, but my mind now produces an ironic "You Were There" documentary, like the famous Walter Cronkite TV series.

My Dad

My father comes to mind first of course, though my memory bank is painfully limited. I lived far away both physically and psychologically during the time he was struggling with MS, being diagnosed in his fifties. I was away from my Stratford, Ontario home, was teaching in BC., in my twenties. I remember how he would have yearly troubles and spend time in hospital, but without a diagnosis. At one point, they performed back surgery. I wasn't in close touch at that point, and was happy to live in an expanding universe outside of the family and small town. My reaction to his illness was, I suppose, quite in keeping with the family approach, which had always been the stiff-upper-lip and backbone school. We didn't talk about illness. I do recall that he was very relieved to be finally diagnosed, to have a name for his problems, after years of tests and doubt.

In those days, I made short, periodic visits home from BC, so saw Dad only occasionally. At that point, he walked with a cane, but I never thought of him as disabled, and can't tell you why. In place of vivid memories, I have a storehouse of guilt and curiosity – what were the invisible symptoms he had to deal with? I remember his feet always being cold, which is a very familiar MS symptom. Did he also have the numbness in his legs that I have? Did he ever experience the bliss of MS euphoria? Did he notice a change in memory and become frustrated with it? What support would he have liked from me?

Grade School

My very first recollection with disability goes way, way back. It must have made a sizeable impact on me, though the details are sketchy. Why else would it still be with me? I was probably in Grade 4 or 5 in my small school in a small town, where there was a boy who used a wheelchair. He had polio, I think. He was younger than me, maybe by a grade or two. I didn't know much about him, and never talked to him; there was certainly no discussion by the teacher in class about what that wheelchair meant. It was his identifying feature as far as we kids were concerned. And it was taken for granted, whatever it might have meant for him or for us. He was like an alien in our midst, but not weird, or frightful – just very different than the rest of us. The teachers obviously missed a wonderful teachable moment, an opportunity to introduce us to a facet of life we hadn't encountered, to expand our view of the world, to develop empathy and understanding. But it's possible that in the early 1950s, the teachers themselves weren't comfortable enough to talk about wheelchairs and disability. So I missed a chance to learn something valuable about life, as did all those students who did not end up needing the insight as much as I did.

Maddie

Maddie was a dear family friend, my mother's age. She had no children of her own and treated my siblings and me very well – did some babysitting and put on the odd party when we were older. And always treats (salted peanuts were my favourite) when we went to visit her and her husband, Harry. She had had some problem as a child which left one leg shorter than the other that caused a severe limp. She always wore special shoes, big black things, unlike those other people I knew wore. But Maddie's disability did not affect her in any way that mattered to a child – she was warm, kind-hearted, generous, and I loved her. She just had funny shoes, that's all. "Very expensive shoes," which is about all I remember her ever saying about them or her walking.

An American Scholar

One year of my undergraduate studies was spent at Laval University in Quebec City. Many students from Canada and the US availed themselves of the French language and literature programs. It was 1967/8, during the Quiet Revolution, as it was called in Quebec, when the province had a prevailing, very anti-English attitude. Though we were there to study the French language and culture, at the undergraduate and graduate level, we were often called "maudit Anglais" (damned English). The atmosphere was tense; the Anglo students ended up socializing together more than any one of us would have liked. The lucky ones quickly found Quebecois boy or girl friends.

One of the students, a middle-aged American woman, walked slowly, with a limp; she too had special shoes. She was doing an MA, and didn't take classes with me, but we were in the same residence. I was as astounded by her being there, carrying on more or less like the rest of us, as people are now when they learn I live alone. She walked slowly, somewhat laboriously; I felt equal amounts of sympathy and impatience. The other thing I remember about her, and can visualize clearly, is her smile. She was very cheerful, which made her more mysterious. She remains someone from my past I would love to talk to, as I learned very little from her about living with a disability and being a minority within a minority. But I did file a vivid picture in my memory. Just being there, in the midst of much younger students, limp and all, she made an impact. I remember her and am grateful for the memory.

The Judge

As a young adult, an overweight woman, I was extremely uncomfortable around swimming pools. But I had always loved swimming and learned to repress the self-consciousness and vanity which would have robbed me of this enjoyable exercise. One very significant 'swim meet' was at the pool of relatives (friends?) of my in-laws in a Toronto suburb. Besides my mother-in-law and the hosts was another guest, a woman somewhat older than me. She arrived with lots of hardware – crutches and braces. She had CP if I remember correctly; in any event, had always been disabled. And there she was, in her swimsuit, carefully divesting herself of all the mobility aids and enjoying a swim with some people she didn't know. Oh yes, she also worked full time . . . as a judge. I saw her only the once, and didn't really talk to her, but I know I learned a lot that day. I couldn't stop staring at her, it all seemed so incongruous –

the swimsuit and the crutches. I owe her a big thank you for providing an image of such resilience.

A Friend with MS

Perhaps the most ironic memory connected with disability is one from 25 years ago or so. A friend from Ontario came out west with a companion. I volunteered to show them the sights, always glad to play tour guide in Vancouver. R's friend, about the same age, had MS, and was using a wheelchair. It was portable and could be collapsed so it fit in the car trunk; we took it out at the viewpoints as we checked out the beauty of Stanley Park, Cypress Bowl, etc. I'm ashamed to admit I remember very little else about her. I do remember my unspoken discomfort, impatience, maybe even frustration with the limitations put on us by the chair. Strangely, given my father's illness, I don't think this experience added to my knowledge or understanding of disability or MS. I was young; I couldn't relate to her situation, didn't know her, didn't know how to talk about her MS, didn't know if it would be all right to ask questions, didn't know, didn't know, didn't know.

As I revisit these memories. I am struck by how unaware I was of the whole topic of disability and how uncomfortable I often felt. But I am also struck by the fact that, in the case of people I really knew, their disability is an adjunct, not the most memorable detail by any means. In fact, the memories did not pop out easily or as a reflex, but had to be researched in my mental disability file. Five contacts with someone with a disability from my childhood or early adulthood, long before I knew anything about anything, much less disability. I wonder if that's about average or if for some cosmic reason I was given more, and was storing those memories to use later.

In 1979, just a few short years after I played tour guide to the woman who had MS, I myself had an attack. Less than two years after that I was diagnosed in China. But it wasn't until 1987 that I started to think seriously about disability. I was using a cane because my balance was poor – but felt a bit melodramatic if I called myself disabled, and fraudulent when I applied for a handicapped parking sticker, as urged by an occupational therapist. It seemed to me, then, that disability was a condition much more serious than my own. Very soon, however, as I depended more and more on the cane, I started watching people who were obviously disabled with greater scrutiny, and wrote of entering a new culture – one I knew little about.

I wasn't horrified as much as confused. And I made mental notes of behaviours, attitudes, approaches – those I liked and those I didn't. Disability became a challenge for me, a study of how to cope, how to do it right. Having been a successful student right through to my MA, I was still looking for top grades, I guess. And having been a teacher all my adult life, it was strange, uncomfortable and humiliating to be so ignorant, so much in need of teachers myself. There have been many who have been models for me. At the same time, I'm thankful for the memories of Maddie, the judge and the others who first showed me disability didn't have to be tragedy. Come to think of it, in my memory bank of disabled people, I am the only one who was uncomfortable.

THE SEVEN DEADLY
ATTITUDES OF MS

*Remember the seven deadly sins? Though they're not at
all deadly and certainly not sins, I have found there are
attitudes which work against me as I cope with MS.
And since my wellness depends on my emotional as
well as physical health, I want to monitor them closely.*

*I know these demons very well, but they may not be
apparent in my e-mail messages; keeping them in check
is one challenge I have to face on my own.*

Control

I believe we can, to some degree, control the course of
our MS. But for someone like myself who has been a
teacher for 30 years, that 'some degree' can be
woefully unacceptable. I get angry, really, really angry when I
have an attack (called an exacerbation) or what is now the
case, a down period. And I think that's because I have trouble accepting my lack of total control over the situation. The
anger is counter-productive and all that negative energy can
be quite toxic.

Vanity

MS has little tolerance for excessive vanity. My balance is poor, yet I refuse to give up walking, so I force myself to walk, at the best of times like someone slightly inebriated ("Poor dear, if she could only see herself."). And if that alone doesn't wear down any vanity I had, the bladder and bowel problems do. Accepting myself as I am now, accepting that I often have little control over many aspects of my appearance, and still feeling good about myself has been a challenge, not a useless one for anyone.

Impatience

Another trait that is far less than helpful. Living with MS requires lots of patience – to accept that it takes longer to do things, for starters. There's usually no need for speed at all (why the rush to hang up my clothes, to make a meal, to write a letter?) so I really must train myself to be calm and accept that I now live life in the slow lane.

Jealousy

After 20 years of living with MS, I would expect this little demon to have completely retreated. Not often any more, but yet once in a while, I find the very negative feeling of envy taking hold. Usually in the summer, when most people's lives expand into the great outdoors. At such times I patiently remind myself that I still have choices, that if this remained a priority in my life, I would still be doing it. It's just not easy anymore, and I can't have everything.

Stubborness

Sometimes it really doesn't hurt to admit I really do need help, that I am not as independent as I like to be. It makes a lot of sense to accept help in matters which are not so vital to me (cleaning, shopping) so I have more energy for the things which are. At my age, I really don't have to prove "I can do it!"

Competition

Old habits die very hard. I know that MS is a very individual condition, that the only comparison that is at all productive is only with myself (was I feeling this way last year at this time? last month? the last time I did so much in one day?) But still I find my competitive side at times comparing what I can or can't do to someone else. I have a serious talk with myself when that happens.

Compulsiveness

Was I always like this? Does it come from having any chronic disease, or specifically MS? Everything takes planning now (combining errands so I need make only one trip, listing the little things I need help with from the homemaker, even planning my moves from one room to another so as to reduce steps). That's all fine and good, probably useful. But when a plan is rigid, when I lose the mental flexibility to adjust 'on the run' I risk creating more emotional toxins. Like when I insist on carrying out my shopping plan (on my scooter) even though it's raining. Like when I am driven to see someone as planned even though I have neither the spirit nor physical energy.

Linda L. Ironside

Demons and emotional toxins do not plague only those with MS or other chronic diseases. Everybody's got 'em – it's part of being human! Yours may not look like mine, which I've lived with for a l-o-ong time. MS has made me much more aware of them and the damage they inflict. But if they think they are in control, they've badly underestimated me; reducing their power is part of my ongoing wellness program.

DIAGNOSIS IN CHINA

Everyone remembers the details of their diagnosis, the tension, the endless tests and the long wait. But few, I expect, remember that process with as much fondness as I do, for I had the good fortune to be teaching in China at the time and diagnosed there.

You will see in part two that in conversations with Flora and Julie I have not dealt in any detail with my diagnosis, as it is clearly one of those how-much-time-have-you-got? topics. This is my description, for them as well as for you. It is taken from notes I made soon after my return to Canada, a year or so after the hospital experience.

n 1979, I had a big yard sale and stored what didn't sell in a friend's basement. I had resigned from a very good job as a consultant with the school board and was heading off to teach in China, at a university in Guangzhou (Canton). I was excited and open to whatever new path life might open in front of me. Luckily, I'd given little thought to the weird symptoms – fatigue, slurred speech – which I'd experienced just a few months before. If I had, I might not have gone.

Once in China, I applied myself in my usual fashion – enthusiastically. I tried to absorb as much of the culture as time would permit. Everything was new to me; my Chinese students and co-workers were themselves enjoying a new openness after the dark years of the Cultural Revolution. I remained on a continual high. I can remember sweeping the floor in my apartment, reflecting on my lack of homemaking interest, and thinking, "Ah yes, but I'm sweeping my floor IN CHINA!"

I was experiencing China the way a typical A personality Westerner does – full out, with no attention to the demands one puts on oneself, either physically or psychologically. I was thrilled to be so involved with my Chinese friends, but cross-cultural communication is not easy; the closer the contact you want, the more stressful it can be. One relationship in particular proved very difficult over the course of the next couple of months. I felt lost, positively adolescent, unsure of what the dynamics of the relationship were, and not aware of just what I should or could do to affect them

My body started to break down just three days after the end of a very stressful trip. I knew something was wrong – constantly tired, sleeping more than usual, but I had arranged to go to Hainan Island, a gorgeous, and at that time isolated island in the South China Sea, to work with the English teachers there. My heart was set on going, so I didn't let on about the fatigue, and honestly believed it would go away in due course. The very first contact I had with the teachers in Haikou, Hainan I was speaking from a podium on a raised platform – turned around to use the chalk board, lost my balance for no apparent reason (poor balance has remained one of my most visible symptoms) and tried to regain it. I can still remember those few seconds of swaying back and forth before I finally fell to the floor. I was embarrassed; my hosts were embarrassed and wanted me to take a break. But I wasn't hurt, and felt better just carrying on. The next few months were to teach me a real respect for the Chinese approach and a mistrust of the North American 'push ahead' attitude when it comes to our health. After I stood up and many hands had brushed me off, I used the teachable moment to make a joke about language teachers having to be willing to make mistakes, to 'fall down'. I was having too much fun to slow down!

It wasn't until I returned to Guangzhou, that things really hit home. One morning, as I was showering, I noticed that I couldn't feel the hot water on my left leg. I'd never been seriously ill, and, at my young age, I couldn't envisage chronic or serious health problems, even when others looked on the situation very seriously. When symptoms continued to develop – trouble walking quickly, constipation – I was given an appointment with a neurologist downtown – as it turned out, a very nervous neurologist. (The responsibility of dealing with a foreigner! And a teacher, at that!)

After some tests at the local hospital, it was quickly decided to send me to Beijing. This wasn't as easy as it sounds. The Foreign Affairs Department in Guangzhou phoned its counterpart in Beijing. They were told to send me with a doctor from Guangzhou who had some contact, or "guanxi", with hospitals in the capital and could "lianxi", a vague term which covers the endless negotiations and diplomatic gymnastics which went on when two work units were involved in one problem. They also chose to send along a young English-speaking Chinese teacher named Liping to act not only as an interpreter, but also as a representative of the university. Her role was to continue the liaison and lianxi after the doctor went home. She stayed with me, in fact, for the duration of the hospital visit, living in the same room with me for most of the following three months.

Linda L. Ironside

Then a stroke of luck. My brother happened to be holidaying in Hong Kong. The visa that could not be issued to him previously was suddenly made available. My joy at seeing him at the university could not match the joy of the doctors, the Foreign Affairs staff involved in my case, or my colleagues: here was the elder brother, who could provide family approval to all the plans, an important step in smoothing my course to treatment in Beijing.

I had tried hard to think of everything I would need in hospital, but of course when I got there, I was ill prepared: no towel, no cup, no soap. The bed presented another problem. I am not extraordinarily tall, about 5'8", but I felt quite the giant as I lay down on the Chinese mattress. It was about three inches shorter than the American bed frame it was sitting on, leaving my head and feet to fall into chasms at either end. A few pillows packed in here and there fixed that up, and I settled in.

Although the medical care I received was superb, there is no denying that the hospital was old, the equipment old, the material standard not as high as I had experienced in Canada. This was not a highly sanitized, sterile, clinical setting. In many ways, it didn't look much like a Western hospital. But some things were the same: the hypos at times felt like blunt swords, the bedpans were slippery and cold, the meals came at ungodly hours. There were good and bad nurses, doctors who should have been car mechanics and others, like my neurologist, who were saints in white. Some nurses were in perpetual existential doubt; others were cheerful Polyannas. One of the main differences from the West was that, in China, medicine was not a business. Doctors did not make money from tests and operations, and were not the elite of the society. They were salaried employees, earning a very modest income, making less than rich peasants on prime agricultural land, less than factory workers lucky enough to top quotas and take home a fat bonus.

Relations between the Chinese staff and foreign patients were much more strained than they were in Guangzhou. Most of the doctors in Beijing were cautious, reserved, and more stiffly professional. This is partially, I think, because of the special status of so many of the "guests", and partially because Beijing, being the seat of power, was generally more tense. The Cantonese, in comparison, seemed more laissez-faire, less worried and reserved. They are China's Southerners, the Californians of that nation. A gregarious Canadian and a gregarious Cantonese presented quite a challenge to the staff in Beijing as we cavorted, sang and joked our way through eleven weeks. It was not easy for both of us foreigners to become accepted, not easy to build a comfortable and casual relationship with most of the doctors and nurses. It was only due to the length of our stay that relations thawed a little and we became well accepted.

The responsibility for foreigners lies very heavy on Chinese shoulders. I was twice a foreigner – not only was I from outside the jurisdiction of the city and the hospital, I was also from outside the entire country. The benefit I gained from this was the thoroughness and the extreme caution on the part of the doctors as they went through their examinations: eyes, ears, nose, throat, insides, outsides, the works. Nothing went unnoticed – my medical records now show that I have an unusually low hairline, front and back, a problem that I found hard to accept at first, but am learning to live with.

The neurologist assigned to me, Dr. Fei, was a small, impish woman who spoke about as much English as I did Mandarin. The pressure on her must have been enormous, but, of course, I saw none of that. She was totally devoted to her work, and I trusted her completely. One example of her kindness and holistic approach was her offer to teach me to knit on her day off, as she was concerned that I was too bored during the weeks of tests leading up to the diagnosis. One of the top neurologists in China offering to teach me to knit – that was hard to get my mind around. Who wouldn't get better with such committed attention and concern?

I benefitted a great deal from the holistic nature of Chinese medicine, which I had heard of but never experienced. It is a lot easier to recover from illness, deal with a diagnosis, or cope with an extended hospital stay when you remain whole, when you never become just a collection of body parts. I was very pleased to know that my emotions were being monitored as well as my physical state. Each morning, Dr. Fei would ask the interpreter, "Jingshen hao bu hao?" ("How's her spirit?"). That simple question each day confirmed for me that I was still being seen as a whole person, and it had a lot to do with the complete faith I had in Dr. Fei.

Once on steroids, I had little crying spells now and again, which I knew were drug-induced. Dr. Fei never stopped recording them. This also served to increase my trust in my doctor, my sense of security, and the feeling that I still mattered as a person. Doctors and nurses did not take over my body, but checked with me about every little procedure. No one said, "We're going to have to . . ." but rather, "Will you accept . . .?" "Can you stand . . .?" They were particularly surprised that I agreed to drink the worst-smelling, most foul-tasting medicine I have ever ingested. "Most Chinese won't take it!" they said, shocked. Years later, when MS was once again quite active in my body, I got advice and a prescription from a TCM (Traditional Chinese Medicine) doctor in Vancouver; once again I agreed to "che ku" to taste bitter, by taking very foul-tasting medicine. A taste, it turns out, I have not yet acquired.

At one point Dr. Fei told me that she wanted to do a spinal tap. This is an unpleasant procedure that involves a needle being inserted into your backbone to withdraw a small amount of spinal fluid. I remembered having one in Canada – the doctor had had trouble inserting the needle and had to try many times; in his frustration, he harshly advised me to lose weight if I ever needed one again. I also remembered my father talking about how horrid this test was. Luckily, MRI (Magnetic Resonance Imaging) scans now render spinal taps unnecessary. When Dr. Fei said she would like to do one and asked if I was willing, I gulped twice – first at the shock of being asked, at her acknowledgement that it was still MY body and second, at the memory of that big, long, nasty-looking needle. But I knew Dr. Fei did nothing lightly and felt safer in her hands than with the diet promoter back home.

I'm glad I agreed, as it turned out to be a fascinating medical experience. She did it right in my hospital room, which reduced considerably the angst of the ride down long corridors and of the operating room. A nurse attended and Liping watched. I was so fascinated by the whole process (pretty well describes my mental state during the whole hospital stay) I didn't work up a bad case of nerves (well, I did in fact have that, but not in the layperson's sense). Dr. Fei's bedside manner made her more of a mother figure than a cold, antiseptic, clinical medical technician. She was quick and proficient. There was little discomfort; I was frustrated only by the fact that Liping was enjoying watching all this, while I could not see it. That took place almost twenty years ago. I've forgotten most details and can't even tell you what was learned from the spinal fluid. But I shall never forget the warm feeling I had through it all, the sense of being secure, cared for, protected.

Another important aspect of healing that I came to understand was the power of time itself. Like most westerners, I viewed my body as something akin to a racecar. Pit stops are rare and brief, with no time for a gradual re-entry onto the track. But the Chinese were not in such a rush – after the diagnosis was made, and I had recuperated for a month, I felt well enough to teach again at the university. The doctors, however, gave strict orders that I was to be allowed to teach only half-time for the next semester, in spite of the fact that I was still getting my full salary. And I later had to admit that my work was more strenuous than I had anticipated. Not going back full time too soon allowed my body to completely recover from the attack and the hospitalization.

At times, however, the pace was frustrating. After a few weeks in hospital, I was getting just a tad impatient, antsy, restless and bored. And my hair was a mess! I have thick, naturally wavey hair; trimming the bush it grows into can be very therapeutic, so I asked if they could have someone cut it. There was a little chatting, and scurrying about, then someone asked the neighborhood barber if he would come into the hospital and do the job. He apparently wasn't sure he was up to cutting the hair of a 'gueilou' (foreigner), so he came over one day to look at my hair and to feel it. This was my first and last audition for a haircut! "Yes," he announced, he would be able to cut it and came back later to do it. Though he'd never met a gueilou before he did an excellent job. Who knows what he thought the hair of a foreigner might be like?

I was in hospital for weeks before Dr. Fei ventured a diagnosis. This delay worked in my favor. She consulted with other specialists as well as the head of neurology at the hospital, and was very thorough in her exploration of my body. She attempted to find every system that was not working as it should be. I was taken to the ophthalmology department for a complete exam, which was, like all the rest, fascinating. I had had surgery for a cataract in one eye, and used one contact lens. One day, Dr. Fei announced with a solemn face, "I have bad news." I can't remember what horror I anticipated, but it was certainly something more frightening than, "You have glaucoma." In my left eye, the one which had had the cataract. Glaucoma, I learned, can result in vision loss if not treated. It was lucky for me that it was caught early and I was started on the eye drops which controlled it before any serious damage.

A fellow ex-patriate in Beijing had loaned me a copy of a medical dictionary, which I read with great interest, the sections on the nervous system and MS in particular. As test after test eliminated other possibilities, I knew that perhaps this was MS, like my father had had. I explained all this to Liping, using the dictionary. "This is beginning to look like something very serious" I told her, and talked about MS and my father. The very next day, a very solemn Dr. Fei came in and announced she and other neurologists who had been consulted had a diagnosis – demylinating disease. Liping cheerfully announced, "Oh, she knows all that!", and told her about the dictionary. The doctor was enraged and grabbed the book from my lap. "She shouldn't know that much" she declared, but realized she couldn't stop me and handed the book back. We had arrived at our diagnosis at the same time, having exhausted other possibilities, both knowing it wasn't a brain tumour as so many had feared. I was told that tales of me perhaps returning to the university in a long, wooden box were circulating at the university.

Dr. Fei was more upset than I was – I was already feeling better than when all this started; my father had had a fairly mild form of MS; I was being well taken care of and continued to draw my full salary. I have never been one to worry too much about what the future might hold.

A number of things made me a very challenging patient for the good doctor. For one thing, I was having a good time, with only short, periodic bouts of depression. One of the more pleasant symptoms of an MS attack is unexplainable euphoria.

It's like a drug-induced high, very nice indeed. I am by nature gregarious; in the hospital I was mentally as well as physically stimulated; Liping and I cavorted like school girls, she exercising none of the humility or reserve more becoming in a Chinese female. On campus in Guangzhou, I knew my extroversion was seen as a little odd, even immature. Children are outgoing, not adults. And here I was in a hospital, in a foreign country, suffering little and seldom acting sickly. Poor Dr. Fei – not only did she have the tremendous pressure of diagnosing this teacher, this foreigner – but of coping with her acting very strangely. The doctor's English was only a little better than my Chinese, although I'd had more exposure to her culture than she to mine. One day I met her in the hall and tried to make a humorous comment, for my own sake as well as hers. She looked up at me (she's short) rather sternly, wagged her finger and announced with a smile, "I think you very childish!" She meant "childlike", of course, and would have been horrified to know how insulting "childish" is to a Westerner.

The tests and medication I was given once MS was diagnosed were very similar to what is used in Canada. One aspect I particularly appreciated was that Dr. Fei never gave me just one type of pill – there was always something given to counteract the side effects common to the primary medication.

Although I was satisfied with the treatment, the Chinese themselves continually apologized for what they thought I must perceive as "backwardness". I fear that if I return to China in twenty years, they'll be efficiently dispensing plastic food on plastic trays, the hospital uniforms will all crackle with starch, music will be piped into every room, machines will monitor a patient's every move, the doctor will make punctual rounds spending five minutes with each patient. And it will be deemed to be modern.

Since the diagnosis turned out to be such a serious, chronic disease, being away from home worked in my favor. There was no one around me fretting, worrying, or despairing as I underwent endless tests in hospital, and no one panicking when the diagnosis was made. On the other hand, there was no one to lean on! I was forced to rely on myself alone to come to terms with my changed reality; I learned that I really could meet the challenges confronting me when I had no other choice.

MS is very rare in the Orient. Consequently, even the people I came into contact with after I got back to home base in Guangzhou did not have an overly melodramatic or negative reaction to the news of my illness. In fact they had either no reaction because they had never heard of the disease or were jubilant that it was not a brain tumor. I had to deal with my own reaction to the diagnosis, no one else's. It's very hard, sometimes, for patients not to take on responsibility for loved ones' sadness or despair. Being removed from people who worried about me, especially people who knew how serious MS can be, helped me remain calm.

The job of getting better was made easier by the financial security I was provided. The last thing you want to have to think about when you're sick is your income or medical bills. I had no such worries since I continued to receive my full salary. When I offered to pay my own plane fare to Beijing, I was told that this was the responsibility of the university. And I didn't have to worry about l losing my job. I felt completely secure, with nothing to think about besides getting better. A very positive mental environment that served me well.

When I got back to Guangzhou, I continued to recuperate in a local hospital. A rather stubborn digestive problem was turned over to a short, elderly, gray-haired, teeth-missing, smiling man who did not look at all like the esteemed Traditional Chinese Medicine doctor he was. He applied three fingers to each wrist, taking the various pulses on which traditional doctors base their diagnosis, told me exactly the symptoms I was feeling, and prescribed what can only be called "forest floor", a cornucopia of flora and fauna which looked like the ground covering of a park in Vancouver without the Coke cans. All manner of elements were there: mineral, vegetable, and animal, each for a specific purpose, some to simply counteract the side effects of the others. Once boiled for a couple of hours in a clay pot, it was given to me to drink. Whether through science, faith, or just good luck, it worked where three months of other medicines had failed.

Compared to Beijing, hospital in Guangzhou was not really much like being in a hospital. I had a large private room with no interpreter in the foreigner's wing, which was an old converted home. Although the neurologist came to see me every day, he did so more for the sake of his English fluency than for any medical reasons. He was truly sorry to see me go home after his five weeks of intensive language practice. Communication with the staff was relatively easy; with only a couple of patients, the nurse on duty and I could often chat away the hours. I too was sorry to go, to leave friends and the most intensive language training I had in China.

Back in Canada more than a year later, I unfortunately slipped back into the North American pace of life as my A personality type resurfaced and I suffered more MS attacks, which left me visibly disabled. Now it's even more important for me, as for all people with disabilities, to do what I can to get the optimum performance from my mind and body. What has stayed with me for twenty years is the understanding I gained in China of health, medicine and my body. My body and mind were empowered to act, as opposed to taking on a passive victim role, which institutionalization often assigns. I have not lost my faith in Chinese medicine, traditional or modern, and still take tablets to help me sleep (no grogginess), to ward off a cold, to balance my hormones. I also get acupuncture treatments, which has helped with a variety of problems, from lack of energy and bladder problems to muscle pain. The irony is that my doctors in Beijing, trained in Western medicine, had told me acupuncture would not help; it was in Canada that I first connected with a Chinese-Canadian doctor, trained in both Western and Traditional Chinese Medicine, who has helped me using acupuncture.

I am still in contact with Dr. Fei, after twenty years. We exchange letters every year at Xmas and occasionally more often. A couple of those letters came from Australia, when she was doing a study sabbatical. When I returned to China to visit friends, five years after I left, I had dinner with her and her family in their modest, comfortable apartment. We're friends the way if often happens – people who have been through something difficult together – in this case, my diagnosis.

Liping, the young teacher who was sent as an interpreter, stayed with me in the hospital until we both went back to Guangzhou three months later. We got along famously and I appreciated her company immensely. Her brother who was living in Beijing came by to visit. Later I got to know the rest of her family in Guangzhou, and had many wonderful visits and meals in their home.

Eventually I came home to Canada and only then thought how nice it would be if Liping had an opportunity to study here. I talked to a prominent Chinese-Canadian, who just happened to be on his way to China, and arranged to meet Liping. He sponsored her, she came, met his bachelor son I did not know, and never left. I was a bridesmaid at their wedding. Liping is now a Canadian citizen and lives with her husband and two daughters in Calgary, Alberta. I've visited them several times. Small world, eh?

Linda L. Ironside

A CHANCE ENCOUNTER

I seldom wrote to both Flora and Julie about the same experience, unless I was asking for advice. I briefly mentioned this chance encounter, but it had such an impact on me it's worth repeating here in more detail.

Outside my small corner supermarket, I noticed a spiffy scooter, obviously parked by someone who had entered the store on foot. I'd never seen it before, nor anyone shopping there who looked as if they might use one, so I wondered whose it might be. I wheeled on in and didn't give it more thought until a well-dressed woman puzzling over the sausages spoke to me, "Oh, I have one of those," she said, looking at my scooter, "but I left it outside. The aisles here are so narrow." She was articulate, friendly, about my age, not at all sick-looking. She stood tall and erect. "Probably not MS. Probably not arthritis," was the script playing in my head as my internal P. I. tried to discern why this woman would use a scooter.

We chatted a bit about our wheels and how we enjoyed them. Eventually we got down to 'brass tacks', when she asked why I needed a scooter. I told l her I have MS, and was happy not to hear the usual reaction to such news – the sudden intake of air, the lowering of the voice and "Oh, dear, I'm so sorry". In fact, she said nothing.

"What about you?" I asked her rather innocently. "Oh, I have Lou Gehrig's disease," she responded very matter-of-factly. Now there was definitely a gulp and a gasp. But I was the one fighting for air; the shoe was on the other foot – I wanted to hug her, to cry, to pity, to patronize, to bemoan. To react the way people do to me, in short – I was just as inept, just as shocked, just as paralyzed. But she didn't allow any of that; she didn't say anything to stop me, but retained her perfect composure, and continued to act like a full human being, not a self-pitying cripple nor heroine. *Less* was *more* in this case.

Wow, what an example to follow! She helped put disability just where I'd like it – a part of life which can't be denied, but it's still only part, and needn't diminish one's dignity.

Linda L. Ironside

HYPO HYSTERIA

This poem was written many years ago, in China, a product of drugs and MS euphoria. I was often awake in the middle of the night, and driven to write.

First the door, it opens only a crack,
Then two little eyes appear.
Smiling at you . . . so friendly,
She really looks like a dear.

Then, just when she's got you smiling,
And thinking the world is fine,
She boldly throws the door open…
Her wicked sneer, a sure sign.

She carries, like a mace before her,
Her weapon, her power, her thrill –
A tray of steel, heavy laden
With what she needs for the kill.

"Should I fight to the death or surrender?
I could put her down with one blow!"
But . . . meekly, I bare what she's after
And grimly brace for the show.

She pretends to be gentle . . . and gently
She dabs at my blue leather thigh.
But needle in hand, she changes.
It's clear she's on a real high.

High up in the air, she holds it,
Then swoops down at once for the kill.
She never fails or misses.
She murmers with glee at will.

Hours later, weak and depleted,
She withdraws all her steel and departs.
Again, there's the smile of an angel –
She's psycho – everyone knows!

I lay on my bed and I ponder,
Make plans for a better defense.
"Give in," I say in conclusion,
"You'll only make yourself tense!

"Your bum is over her barrel,
There's nothing you can do.
So grin and bare it, be cheery
And get used to being blue!"

Linda L. Ironside

FATIGUE AND MS

*Fatigue is my most troubling symptom of MS, one I
mentioned a lot in e-mails to Flora and Julie. This is a
tad more rational than the rants in Part Two; it is an
article I first wrote years ago when MS was new to me;
it remains an accurate description.*

"Boy, oh boy, I'm so tired I could just drop!" Everyone has
had fatigue at one time or another; you're at the end of
your rope, physically or mentally, or both and you just
can't go on, no matter how much you want to.

The difference between that and the kind of fatigue I get
with MS is that healthy people don't actually drop – they can
push themselves if they absolutely must. They feel as if they
can't go on, but actually drop only when finished whatever it is
that put them in that state; the election campaign or the kids'
party or Christmas, the overtime at work has ended, the three
people in the family they've been nursing for the past week are
all over the worst, and the last assignment for the course
they've been taking is off to the typist.

I can't – go on, that is. I don't even really get advance
warnings; mine is not a gradual wearing down. My body or
mind or both just stop. In the middle of a conversation or a

meeting, an overwhelming wave of fatigue can wash over me so completely that I can continue only as a passive listener; I've had trouble having enough energy to just follow.

"Fatigue," since it's a word used to describe the tiredness all people feel at one time or another doesn't really catch it. There just isn't a better word for it, however, which I regret, since it is the most insidious symptom of a most fickle and insidious disease. The language is deficient and we have to settle on the word at our disposal.

On the larger scale, 'fatigue' means I sleep 8-10 hours a day, have a nap or a rest at least once a day, and plan my days with it in mind. That's when I'm feeling my best; during an exacerbation, or relapse, I can sleep 12 hours a day for weeks. Every person with MS has, in some ways, a different case, though, so we must be careful not to make too many general-izations. There seems to be no definitive picture.

Marathons, in a wheelchair, on a bike, or with a prosthesis, have become a popular way for the disabled to proclaim their abilities to a world that may have exaggerated their disability. But stories of such feats by people with MS may be giving people the wrong message. Physical accomplishment for us is not a matter of drive, or push, or physical prowess, as much as it is, surely, a matter of good management, good planning and recognition of the particular nature of the disability. A person with MS in a wheelchair is not another Rick Hansen, nor should they be seen as someone who could be. MS is not a disability in an otherwise healthy body; it isn't the result of an accident; it's a disease of the central nervous system whose symptoms are as extensive and pervasive as that system itself.

The recognition that is given those who exert themselves, push their bodies and endurance to the limits, join the fitness revolution can be a problem for people with MS. Before I had any visible symptoms, and was still working, my colleagues did not know there was anything preventing me from joining in. Not only did I have to deal with the fatigue; I also had to deal with the guilt I felt when I opted out of social events, or when I took the easy way out. (As with most guilt, this came not just from pressures around me, but also from my own head.) It's easier now, using a cane, which provides mental as well as physical relief – I now have a problem which is in essence not much different than it was, but now it's visible. Gone are the joking enquiries about why I take the elevator in favor of the stairs; gone is the need for excuses about my "bad knee", which prevented my participating in the square-dancing. It seemed at the time that some explanation was called for – I chose the 'bad knee' because that kept me in the fitness club; people get bad knees from skiing, or jogging, or aerobics class when they're over-exuberant. Bad knees give you more status in the fitness-oriented world.

I've learned to budget energy as carefully as I do my money. My goal is to have 'money in the bank' for the things that I want to do most, and not let it dribble away walking up a flight of stairs when an elevator is available, or standing in line or doing the myriad of little errands and tasks that used to require only my time and patience, not my valuable livable life. I have learned how to be energy conscious, an efficiency expert in energy conservation. Good advice was provided by physiotherapists, occupational therapists, and the MS Society, which makes available a plethora of printed materials – how to prepare low-on-energy meals, how to organize your home to reduce steps required, how to manage a job so you'll not only get it done, but have some "money" left over for a little life afterward.

A very sensible and sensitive O.T. persuaded me years ago to get a disabled sticker for the car, so that I could take advantage of parking that's close to entrances. I occasionally still

have the urge to explain to people who see me, a too-young-
for-a-cane and seemingly healthy woman, about my legs and
how important it is for me to be kind to them. I can stand or
walk only for twenty to thirty minutes, and treat this limited
energy like gasoline in my car – I make sure I leave home with
a full tank, but know it's limited and I can't get more until I get
home again, so don't squander it.

When a person's body is crying for rest, for a little TLC,
they don't think the idea of staying in bed all day Sunday is a
burden or a hardship, even when the sun is shining and the day
is inviting others to get outside and enjoy it. When you feel
that tired, going to bed is not a problem.

So, too with me – the cane, the sticker, the attention paid
to energy quotas do not represent a problem, but a solution.

NOT EXACTLY
"PUTTING ON A TOP HAT"

Julie, Flora and I talk about our various mobility aids – canes, walkers, scooters, forearm crutches. Those conversations inspired me to have a little fun with the topic of my ineptitude with a cane, though I never admitted this failing to them.

Being disabled is not much of a problem on my scooter. In fact, it can be fun, passing able-bodied walkers on the sidewalk with a friendly little beep. Showing off for young children, who are always enthralled with what must look to them like a super toy.

My cane, though – now, that's another story. I used to associate a cane with Fred Astaire, so nimbly drifting across my screen. (Of course, he was using a walking stick, but in the eyes of a child, it was a cane.)

Later I watched the elderly gentleman down the street going for walks on sunny and not-so-sunny afternoons, always with his cane. He walked purposely, strode actually, back straight, eyes clearly fixed on something just ahead. He didn't use his cane as much as flourish it. It was an accessory, part of the image he created on the street. I couldn't imagine him without it.

What a disappointment it was, therefore, when I started to use a cane myself. And still now, years later, I have failed to capture the Fred Astaire look – the grace, the artistry, the flair. They both made it look so easy, Fred and the dignified neighbour. But it turns out it's not all that simple. I don't walk tall. I lean. I wobble. And I still occasionally plant the cane firmly on someone else's foot or whack a person on the shin (crowds are a challenge). All in all, the world's a much safer and lovelier place with me on my scooter rather than prowling around with a big stick.

The problem is not the cane itself; it's my hands, namely the fact that I have only two. The cane takes one, leaving only one for the many, many things I cannot do with my teeth, knees or other parts of my body which occasionally hold things. Like getting in the car in the morning. With a purse, keys, cane, and maybe a briefcase, I am completely overwhelmed by baggage, more like a world traveler than a woman off to tutor a student. What does one do with a cane while unlocking a car door? At that point, it's just a long nuisance. No one needs a cane to open a car door; what one needs is hands, of which I find myself in short supply. I've tried leaning the cane against the car, and stretching my free hand so it alone can take care of purse and briefcase. I have even placed the cane on the ground or on the roof for a moment, but that seems to lack a certain je ne sais quoi.

I invariably end up using a tactic I call the BPM or Body Pressure Maneuver. It's simple enough, if a bit lacking in the style department. I sandwich the cane between my body and the car, leaving one hand free to hang on to the baggage and the other to do the key work. That is, if I have remembered to make my 'sandwich' on the back door, leaving the front door accessible. I wonder how the man down the street did it?

Linda L. Ironside

Another place I always run out of hands is a cafeteria. I watch young kids deftly carrying their tray in one hand, and fishing for money with the other. How do they find the centre of gravity? They can't all be physics students. Maybe I just eat the wrong kind of foods, a little on the heavy side – sadly, I cannot carry my tray with one hand, and again, I find I have just too much baggage (tray, wallet, cane) for only two hands.

The scooter is definitely classier, more appealing. It has wheels and is motorized – a big attraction with anyone over the age of two. A cane, on the other hand, tends to make people think of ski accidents and hospitals. But for me, it will always be the image I have failed so miserably to recreate – Fred Astaire, complete with top hat.

THERE, BUT FOR
THE GRACE OF GOD

No one with MS would ever say it's easy or a blessing. But Flora, Julie and I recognize simply, that it is a not insurmountable part of life. I take that a bit further.

I've had MS for twenty years. In that period of time, I've gone through periods of denial, anger, depression and suicidal loneliness. But finally I've reached a place of peace about this disease; on a good day, I can even think about what life would have been without it and say, "There but for the Grace of God, go I."

MS is, at times, a heavy burden to carry. What other disease would leave me with mobility, balance, bladder, and cognitive problems and at the same time take away the energy needed to deal with it all. But on a good day, I remind myself, I might never have encountered disease at all, and remained in the state of innocent ignorance I see in so many others. I might never have experienced the personal growth which MS has afforded me. I remember the valuable lessons I've learned in the past twenty years.

There are people who suffer from good health, for whom illness is a terrifying insult, or who have never learned to accept

Linda L. Ironside

physical losses and problems as they age. I shall never be, like others I know, shocked and embittered by the aging process. Neither will I be intimidated by doctors or surrender my health to others.

And in the meantime, while I'm still "young", I get to wear comfortable shoes with impunity, I get to say "No" when I never allowed myself to before. I get to look after myself without feeling guilty, a rare luxury for women. "I've gained as well as lost", I say to myself on a good day. On bad days, of course, it can still look like a pretty raw deal.

Without MS, I would never have ventured into counseling, which has put a mirror in front of me such as nothing ever did before. I might never have ventured out of the comfortable middle class, never have had a look at marginalized people in my society or have felt the sting of it, never have learned to empathize. I would never have been motivated to look into alternative therapies, which have helped with more than MS.

On a CBC radio program in February of 1997, Oliver Sachs, the real life doctor behind the film, "Awakenings", spoke of working on the island of Guam. "They treated disease as . . . part of life," he observed. MS has allowed me to treat disease, not as an aberration, not as an ugly monster, but rather a "part of my life", like adolescent zits, aging and the death of loved ones. This may sound too Polyanna to be credible, but it sure beats the heck out of being angry all the time.

IT'S ALL ABOUT ATTITUDE

You have probably figured out by now that I am a pathological optimist, which is my good fortune. I know a good attitude is more than just wishing to have one. The following is a reflection I did for the MS Society Bulletin on this important, yet puzzling topic.

t's all about attitude, that helps a lot," is something I hear often. And there's more and more being written on the mind/body connection to convince us that our mental attitude is a big part of our wellness. It is in our best interest to maintain a healthy attitude. But what exactly is a good attitude? Is it the same for all people? Does it simply represent a certain personality type, i.e. the optimist? Can everyone achieve it?

Maybe a good attitude means no special attitude, just carrying on with your life. Maybe a good attitude means acknowledging the disease but not staring at it – not being consumed, controlled, owned by the disease any more or any longer than we are by any of life's events. This does not mean denying we have a serious illness and that mobility, bladder, bowel problems, memory loss, balance difficulty, vision loss, spasms, etc., can be extremely difficult at times. But with time and patience, maybe even MS can be put in perspective, and not be given any more power in our lives than necessary. Of course, it changes us. But does it have to rob us of our very essence?

We had no choice in getting this disease, but we are still masters of how we react to it. We didn't choose what is on our plate, but we can choose what condiments to eat with it. We still have choices to make!

You recognize a good attitude the moment you encounter it. I recently met a middle-aged woman who had suffered a major stroke a few years ago, and after a long struggle, had come to terms with her disability. She now used forearm crutches, and one eye was partially affected, so she was no longer able to drive. Yet she smiled easily, participated fully in family events, and said to me that in some ways she enjoys life more now than she did pre-stroke. How can that be?

She explained that she appreciates life on a different level now, a deeper level. I think the quantity of her enjoyment has perhaps not changed, but the source of it has. When life gets serious, you no longer have time for living only on the surface. Makenna is a wonderful woman, and I was pleased to meet her and her attitude.

Are we who have MS so different from people without it? Who gets through this life without struggle, without being tested at least once to the very core? Is MS harder than losing a child because of a drunk driver? Harder than having no money to provide a proper life for your children? Harder than watching a loved one waste away with cancer? Harder than having one of the invisible mental conditions which can be socially debilitating and so little understood? I wonder.

The smaller the challenge, the harder it hits, it seems. We all know people who seem to have no reason for anguish at all, who fall to pieces over a minor car accident, a downturn in the market, who cannot cope with the fact that they are getting older. We would gladly change places and challenges, but in their world, they are also having a very hard time. My good attitude about having MS tells me not to lose compassion for others whose problems look so small to me. After all, People with MS (PwMS) don't have a corner on suffering.

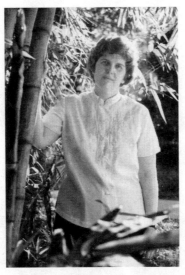

This picture was taken in Guangzhou, in a bamboo grove
on the campus of Zhongshan University.

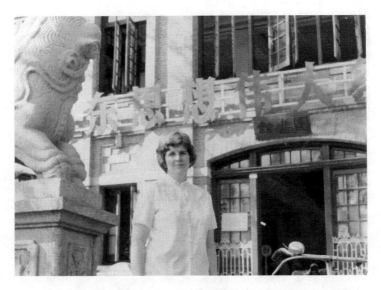

China, 1980 – in front of a sign extolling the virtues of Mao.

Sharing MS

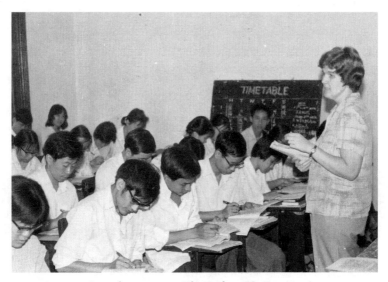

In a classroom at Zhongshan University,
Foreign Languages Department.

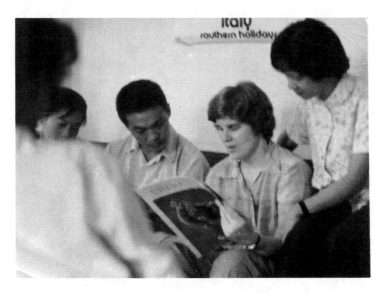

With students in my apartment, Zhongshan University, 1979.

Linda L. Ironside

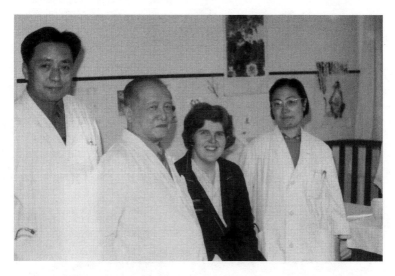

Three neurologists in my room at Capital Hospital,
Beijing, China, 1980.

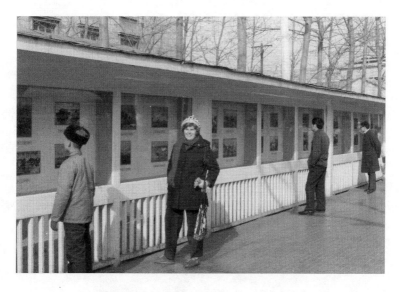

The streets of Beijing, December 1980.

Sharing MS

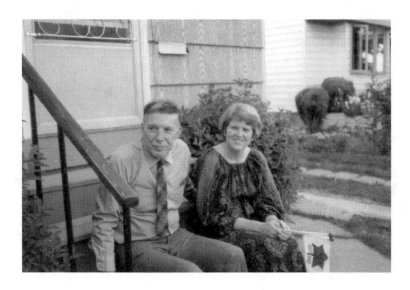

My father and I on the front steps of the family home, 1976.

Sharing
MS

PART TWO ~ MS CHAT

WELCOME

$\mathcal{W}$elcome to this print version of e-mail to and from my MS cyberbuddies. The atmosphere here is warm and friendly, so pour yourself a coffee, pull up a comfortable chair and get to know our little group. Flora and I live in the same city, so our cybertalk is sometimes supplemented by phone calls. In contrast, I first met Julie on the Internet, though we did later meet in person. We're all sharing with you bits of our e-mail letters. You will see that, although we have certain symptoms and treatments in common, each one is unique in their experience of the disease. Par for the course with MS.

There's never a good time to have a chronic illness. But there could be a worse time than now, when we can be connected electronically to people all over the world; my MS community stretches from every province in Canada to the U.S. and Britain, on to Europe and Africa. So many people all over the world sharing their frustrations with the disease and often as well, their continuing delight with life. Julie, Flora and I could never have shared so much with pen and paper correspondence, given the limitations MS puts on us. I wouldn't even have met Julie were it not for the Internet. We met through Jooley's Joint, www.mswebpals.org, a web site for PwMS. One of those wonderful services you find here and there on the Net – this one matching people, like pen pals. It was a blind date, which paid off big time.

I've been e-mailing Flora and Julie for more than two years. However, this section is not organized chronologically, but by broad themes picked from the library of our messages. Things change over two years in anyone's life and even more so in the case of PwMS. As you read, you may find that something is said at one point which is expanded upon later (change of drug protocols, for example) or even contradicted. Along the way, I decided to use a walker, Flora decided to have grandchildren, Julie decided to switch drugs. And by the time this gets to print details will no doubt have changed again.

It should be stated, too, that there have been times when our writing has been interrupted by the course of the disease. Often this is mentioned in our e-mail; sometimes it is not. The book is a distillation of our correspondence, rather than a mere recording of it. Throughout, I've tried to give you an honest description of our lives with MS, complete with the fluctuations.

THE WRITERS

Flora, Julie and I share one of the most common symptoms, trouble with walking. But there's a myriad of other symptoms, some we share and some not, to varying degrees, and at varying degrees. Getting confused? It's hard to put your finger on the disease; it's very individualized – there are no absolutes in either symptoms or reactions. For example, of the three of us, only Flora has to deal with serious vision problems. All, at one time or another, have experienced the peculiar nerve fiber fatigue which results from the fact that nerve connections (synapses) are not made easily and the nerves need a rest. And of course we can all talk about the changes, frustrations, and challenges of living with a chronic disease and a disability. But most important, we have all learned how to live with MS and not be a victim of it. Our mutual support has been a big help in that. Here are a few details on your writers, in their own words.

Flora McLeod

I had my first symptoms in 1992 when I was fifty-five years old. I also had eye problems ten years earlier which where diagnosed as macular degeneration and not MS. This is still a subject of disagreement between neurologists.

However, my diagnosis in 1994 was a relief (at least I wasn't dealing with a brain tumor). Actually, the first suggestion of what the symptoms meant came in 1992 from a trusted naturopath. I was working, of course, and happily saw the numbness simply go away after a few weeks. That was before I had learned about relapsing remitting symptoms. And life went on: acquiring a lovely island home and acreage, traveling to the UK (holiday), Europe (international conference) and Hawaii (Christmas trip with our children), my daughter Claire's wedding in Sweden. My work was going fine including a reprint of a book I had published, taking on the presidency of a child advocacy group and the move of my work place to a new location. I continued my interest in social planning, adult education, children's advocacy, and writing.

The symptoms were mild and manageable, including reduced vision in one eye, but my extensive gardening and travel every weekend was not something I could maintain. So my husband and I moved to a house nearby my work at the new Justice Institute in New Westminster. Not having a daily commute to Vancouver or a weekly one to the island was a help and I focused on the new garden, doing more planning and management than heavy work. And on the job, things progressed at their usual hectic pace. I took a trip to Oxford,

Cambridge and Glasgow with Claire in the summer and became aware of the need for safety and the use of a cane.

Three months later, in 1996, an exacerbation changed everything over the course of a weekend, when I left work and drove home for the last time.

Walking problems had worsened rapidly: use of my right hand was difficult and eye sight had deteriorated, with blurred vision in what had been my good eye to result in general low vision.

Currently, I am mobile in protected settings but use a wheel chair on the street or in a store or mall. I have yet to decide on a scooter or other mobility aid, the decision being complicated by the eyesight problem.

Yes, blind people get across roads, but not usually on a scooter! While I have low vision, I still read with adaptive lenses and the book, magazine or newspaper held a couple of inches from my nose. The expression "a heavy book" I take literally – too heavy is just plain tiring.

I used e-mail at work as well as a listserve connection, so when I began to spend my time at home, the continuation of an e-mail contact was most welcome. I also bought a 19 inch monitor and have upgraded my computer to take advantage of the new technology. I can read the screen without magnification or even glasses so using computer e-mail is a delight.

I have three adult children and a stepchild and more recently two grandchildren who along with their parents are much in touch with me in spite of living in different countries. Electronic mail plays a big role. In fact, I saw the first photos of my grandson, Adrian, on the internet.

I took a trip to New York 1997 before my granddaughter, Rue, was born and I flew to Stockholm last year to visit Claire's family. Adrian was then 17 months old but I plot and plan constantly about the next major trip. Recently Sarah and Rue were here renewing contact with us and with Adam, my son, and their popular uncle.

I am in my sixties and live on Long Term Disability (LTD) and pension. I have recently moved to a location nearer friends and family, which will give me more freedom for relatively independent living.

Julie Zuby

I am a "Michigander", which is what those of us residing in Michigan, USA call ourselves. My husband, Mike, and I live in a suburb of Detroit, Farmington, and have lived here for almost twenty years. My life is good, although when I say that to some people, there is usually a need to explain the statement. New people, upon meeting me, see at least one of my assorted mobility aids, and from that observation, make negative assumptions about the quality of my life. Challenges and bad days, sure, and many of them, but MS has actually given me a much heightened sensitivity to the wonderful people and circumstances around me. Would I banish MS from my life if I could? In a heartbeat! But, I can't! So, it seems right to enjoy life by seeking people, tools and other accommodations to facilitate access to all the good stuff. It's the cup-is-half-full thing in my nature that allows me to do that, and I am truly thankful for that philosophy.

I worked for almost thirty years in health care. My career began as a Registered Respiratory Therapist and advanced over time through to various roles in supervision, education, and ultimately administrative responsibility for several patient care departments. MS wasn't willing to allow me to continue in that direction and I had to retire in 1997 due to my disability.

I was diagnosed in 1993 at the ripe old age of fifty-one, after developing frightening symptoms while I was overseeing a large public event at the hospital on a very hot day. My right leg wasn't working and I was experiencing a loss of balance. I retreated twice to my office and lay down on the floor to recover and think. All I did was become more frightened.

This started me down the diagnosis trail. Medical people have a tendency to draw conclusions based on their exposure to large sources of information and experience with patients. I approached my physician with a not-so-well-received statement, "I think I have MS" to which he said, "Who is the doctor here?" Deep down, I hoped that that it was MS because secretly, I thought I had a giant brain tumor. I think I was fortunate in that based on historical recollections of mine and my doctor's aggressive use of diagnostic tools, Magnetic Resonance Imaging, spinal tap, evoked potential studies, etc., I was only in limbo for about ten months. My neurologist confirmed my introductory statement the following July.

My family is wonderful. I am married to the greatest guy … husband, lover, father, grandpa, and best of all, my closest friend. Michael is an engineer, working for a sunroof manufacturer. He is liaison between his company, the auto design staff and manufacturing functions. He has a few years to work before we plan to retire in a place with warmer winters.

My adult daughters are also close friends, and I love them dearly. Darlene is married to Jeff; they are the parents of David and Daniel, three year-old twins. Cheryl, her sister, one year younger, is married to Bruce. They are mom and dad to a six year-old boy, Cole, his four and a half year-old brother, Logan, and Karlee, who will soon be three. Karlee does her best to make her mark in the male-dominated club of siblings and cousins. They will never think of her as easy to push around. They are, of course, a source of great joy to Mike and me. This great family, along with some very good friends, make every day one for which I am grateful.

Linda L. Ironside

Linda Ironside (your humble guide):

I introduced myself in Part One – diagnosis at age 33, now disabled, retired from a career in education, divorced, no children. MS has given me time to indulge in my favourite pastime, writing. It has also given me much to think and write about.

In this book, I divulge much more about myself than I originally thought such a project would require; that too has encouraged me to stretch and grow. No point saying more; you're sure to draw your own conclusions about who I am from these pages.

THE WRITERS CHAT

I know a lot of people with MS and know of many more: friends, acquaintances, a relative, friends of relatives. But I haven't talked to anyone about their life with MS as much as I have with Flora and Julie.

They are amazing women, who have inspired and encouraged me. I have enjoyed sharing my life with them and being given the privilege of hearing about their lives.

Three women with MS, their computers and a love of e-mail – we have a lot in common, a lot to share. Flora and Julie are intelligent women who have found a way to cope with the disease and fashion a quality of life. But I like to hear about more than their MS. Like their joy with the grandkids, who just happen to also be grand kids, I'm told, and the consulting work each is still doing, and the trips they go on and well, you'll see.

FLORA

*Flora and I met through a mutual friend who felt we
had a lot in common. We now both live in Vancouver,
but did not when we first met. We enjoy the flexibility
of communicating by e-mail (communicating only
when we feel alert and without stress) although we
occasionally also have phone chats. Flora is one of my
many friends with MS, the one I have shared the most
with pertaining to MS because we quickly began enjoying our e-mail correspondence.*

Flora to Linda:

I was so glad we met the other day. It's a huge bonus to me to
talk with another person with MS and who likes to keep in
touch via e-mail. An additional bonus – you have the skill to
help me with my rather mundane e-mail or other computer
problems.

As I briefly explained, I was diagnosed in 1994 after having
first symptoms two years earlier. These receded over the next
month then cleared completely meaning that I made no
lifestyle changes. I continued to work as usual as a Program
Director at the Justice Institute of BC where I had been happily
employed for ten years. After a confirmed diagnosis, I did try
to simplify life, cutting back travel, reducing rather extensive
gardening and a range of chores, but not much in the light of
what I had to do once my first major exacerbation struck. This
happened five years after those first symptoms when I was
fifty-nine years old. I was in shock. In the course of one weekend my walking became difficult, my right hand was crippled

beyond use for several months and my eyesight deteriorated rapidly. I parked my car in the drive for the last time. I went on short term disability for six months and then long term disability at which point my income was reduced nearly to half.

Major trauma! My husband, Alan, who works from home, therefore took on all the marketing. (I was not mobile and couldn't see very well.) He found himself doing all the cooking for the same reasons while continuing his own work. What a lifestyle shift for us both – "exacerbated" by my not being able to get down the basement stairs to do laundry, manage much of anything in the garden or get away from the house on solo trips. Of course he had worked from home before, but I had never in our relationship, been present so consistently or needing so much care and assistance. Role reversal was quickly, and it seemed permanently in place.

Long term disability meant facing the possibility or even reality of not working again, giving up my rather nice office and feeling the close connections I had at work gradually pulling apart.

Also, I was facing the fact that our home would no longer do. Steps down to the front door, many steps up to the back door and a tricky set of stairs all around the house. All this made for a wonderful view but a flood of limitations in existing in a rather pleasant place.

But not walking well and not driving meant a sudden end to my independence. No going to work of course, traveling, making my own decisions or being able to plan my life. And not just for me but for my family. From being the one who did so much, enjoyed so much and being the glue that held things together (including a well-defined role in our financial affairs), the ground shifted dramatically. So, the long struggle to regain parts of my independence and accepting the help I need began.

Linda L. Ironside

What were your initial losses and the shifts in what constituted life for you? Even more important, where and how have you rebuilt?

Linda to Flora:

What a big, big question – because I have largely rebuilt my whole life in the last ten years, since MS really became a factor. I'll save my story of diagnosis (in China) for a separate slow news day, and try to concentrate on what you asked. I was diagnosed in 1980, but didn't suffer much until 1986-7 when I had four attacks in one year, ending up in a group home, disabled, and depressed. The biggest loss for me was the loss of self. Where was the happy-go-lucky, easy-going Linda I knew? Where was her smile? I would stand in front of the mirror and see if the smile muscles and brain patterns still could work together to produce something that looked real. I thought my life as I had know it, was over; I wished it was. Being alone, although it felt awful at the time, was actually a benefit. I had to keep working (keep pretending I was competent, though I no longer reached my old measure of ability in the classroom), so I just went through the motions, and tried to find medical, psychological help along the way. A counselor helped me a lot; the drugs I was prescribed, however, made my loss of self more acute; I felt as if I were living life through an opaque curtain, not really in touch with anything. Gradually, I got better and Linda re-emerged. Going on LTD in 1995 seemed like a very natural thing to do – carrying on was such a struggle, and my life consisted of little more than preparing classes and teaching them. Even though post depression I had renewed spirit, MS still limited my energy and concentration. In retrospect, my life has been an hourglass. Started out wide and full and vibrant, then got very, very small for a while. And now it's full again, with new challenges, new stimulation, new discoveries, new acceptance of MS and its place in my life. This end of the hourglass looks quite different than the other one, but the basic structure is the same, the chemical make-up, the size. I've learned a lot, and actually value this end of the glass a lot. Have you ever done the exercise of listing the positives in your life which resulted from MS? It's important for me to do this, as it is proof that the optimistic, cheerful, smiling Linda still lives here.

For most people, MS means Microsoft. For Flora, Julie and me, it means a lot of different things, not just Multiple Sclerosis. We have had fun coming up with all the names those letters could stand for.

Flora to Linda:

Trying to remember a conversation we had on names for MS. Do you have a list? When one doesn't complain eloquently enough or gives in to some medical person's belief it's not so bad – Misguided Stoic.

Linda to Flora:

> Misguided Skeptic
> Miserable Sneak
> Mega Shit (a contribution from a member of an MS
> newsgroup)
> Mystery Show
> Mean SOB
> Multiple Stories
> Many Sores, Spots
> Mucho Serious

Flora to Linda

I am recalling your comments around Thanksgiving Day last October. I liked your way of saying that a good day was one in which our disease (or disability) did not dominate. But I find there are ways disability can be appraised from another and friendly perspective.

I have another baby in my life now as well as the two grandchildren who were both just two years old last month but who both live in distant and different cities. The new child, Moses, is about eleven months old and here in Vancouver. He visits with his mom who works with me on occasion – shopping, sorting my desk, organizing my files so I can find things I put away in spite of the low vision situation. She is a prime factor in reducing my frustration level.

Bu what I have appreciated about Moses is a repeat of the frank look of uncomplicated, unbiased interest he gave when he noticed me using a walker. "Wow! I would like one of those!" was his expression. Both Adrian and Rue, the children of my other daughter, had had the same look at varying times. And, a little older, got hands-on experience in running it about. They seemed to understand adult concern about safety and showed their skill at braking, climbing safely and particularly being willing to return it to 'Gamma' if she needed it. A repeat of that appraising and approving glance was nice to see.

I am in the process of deciding if I can make use of either a scooter or power chair with the help of at least two physio-therapists. If I do decide on one, wait till the little kids see that! My concern is not so much the low vision problem which certainly does concern Alan, as whether or not I will become too dependent. "Think freedom and independence" I tell myself. And adaptability. But that's all part of more and new future good days as well.

When I first started using a cane, I didn't immediately think of myself as disabled. My life was going on pretty well as before, just that I felt more secure using a cane. "Do eyeglasses make someone disabled?" I asked. "And who cares who is and who isn't disabled?" It turns out doctors care . . . and insurance companies care . . . and the government cares. There's a need for a common language when speaking about disability, the severity and extent. But both Flora and I have concerns about the scale presently in use in Canada.

Linda L. Ironside

_____

Linda to Flora:

Have you had a chance to look at/think about the scale which is used to define a person's level of disability? I've heard about this thing, the KDS (Kurtzke Disability Scale) but never actually seen it until someone on the news group posted it. I was very curious . . . at first, wondering if I was a:

> 4.5 – fully ambulatory without aid, up and about much of the day, able to work a full day, may otherwise have some limitations of full activity or require minimal assistance; relatively severe disability; able to walk 300 meters without aid.

But how could I tell? Does a cane count as aid? And work a full day at what? What I used to do or anything? What counts as work? Maybe I'm a:

> 5.0 – ambulatory for about 200 meters, disability impairs full daily activities.

Then I tossed the whole concept in my mental trash bin. Apart from the vagueness and ambiguities, how would one "work a full day" if one wasn't "up and about much of the day"? This probably makes sense to the neurologists; they're no doubt clear on what it means. But it is still far from able to give an accurate picture of my disability, or anyone else's, as far as I am concerned. Same old problem with conventional medical practice – it's not holistic and people are. Level of disability has as much to do with emotions and spirit as with legs. And in our (MS) case, even the leg thing is not constant. Since there's no criteria in the scale which deals with stability of level or ability, it doesn't work well for me. In fact, it makes me a little annoyed to see these levels all spelled out, with no consideration to anything but the physical side of life – and even that, not very thoroughly (missing the fluctuations possible, writing it as fixed and consistent).

If my spirit is strong, my legs are more able than on days when I feel unmotivated and down. MS is surely a disease where the mind/body interplay is of great importance. So, I wonder, just what does anyone do with this scale which does not give the full picture? How does it help any medical professional?

For your information, Flora, here it is:

The Kurtzke Disability Scale (KDS)

The KDS is a scale designed to follow overall course of a disease outcome or treatment. There is a correlation between the Kurtzke Functional System (KFS) rating system and the Expanded Disability Status Scale (EDSS).

KDS value or degree of disability in detail:
- 0   normal neurologic exam
- 1.0   no disability, minimal signs on one FS
- 1.5   no disability, minimal signs on more than one FS
- 2.0   minimal disability in 1 FS
- 2.5   minimal disability in 2 FS
- 3.0   moderate disability in 1 FS; or mild disability in 3-4 FS, though fully ambulatory
- 3.5   fully ambulatory but with moderate disability in 3-4 FS
- 4.0   fully ambulatory without aid, up and about 12 hrs/day despite relatively severe disability; able to walk 500 meters without aid

4.5   fully ambulatory without aid, up and about much of the day, able to work a full day, may otherwise have some limitations of full activity or require minimal assistance; relatively severe disability; able to walk 300 meters without aid

5.0   ambulatory for about 200 meters, disability impairs full daily activities

5.5   ambulatory for 100 meters, disability precludes full daily activities

6.0   intermittent or unilateral constant assistance required to walk 100 meters with or without resting

6.5   constant bilateral support required to walk 20 meters without resting

7.0   unable to walk beyond 5 meters even with aid, essentially restricted to wheelchair, wheels self, transfers alone

7.5   unable to take more than a few steps, restricted to wheelchair, may need aid in transfer, wheels self but may require motorized chair for full day's activities

8.0   essentially restricted to bed or chair or perambulated in wheelchair, but may be out of bed much of day, retains self-care functions, generally effective use of arms

8.5   essentially restricted to bed much of day, some effective use of arms, some self care functions

9.0   helpless bed patient, can communicate and eat

9.5   unable to communicate or eat/swallow

10.0 death

Mmmm, I never thought of 'death' as a level of disability before. That's almost funny; I can laugh at it because I know MS does not progress like that. What do you make of all of this?

I sure hope it doesn't rain for too long – I'm going on a boating trip soon, and seven days on a boat in the rain would render MS the least of my problems, I'm sure. Compared to insanity, suicide, homicide . . . .

Have a good week on land.

Flora to Linda:

I suppose the scale is an attempt at objectivity. I agree that the interpretation of what disability means to an individual is a most subjective matter. The reference under 7.5 to a full days activities is bemusing. It raises questions about how fatigue is defined and evaluated and of course, what the activities are. Are they stressful in an emotional sense? If the test involved, say, giving evidence in court for a full day, a motorized chair may not do the trick.

I am curious that use of hands is not included as a distinctive disability measure. Is it assumed to be the same as effective use of arms? And there is no reference to eyesight. From my experience, the inability to see clearly affects how effectively I can use my hands or arms and how able I can be in walking.

JULIE

Julie started as my cyber-pal, a woman I 'met' on the Internet. It's quite amazing and quite wonderful how quickly she and I became virtual, and then real world friends. Our e-mails were easy and fun right from the get-go. But then, you can judge that for yourself.

Linda to Julie:

It's a rainy day here, well suited to sitting at the computer and day-dreaming. Thinking up things I don't know about you. Don't go getting all nervous on me, now; my questions are mild and innocent.

Like, how much connection do you have with other people with MS, the so-called MS community? Are you a member of any newsgroups? I belong to three different ones to do with MS, but only one is very active. I like the anonymity of the groups, although I do know the local people who are members. I appreciate getting a broader view of MS than just my own and my friends' cases. Like, being reminded of the pain which many people have as a result of MD. (That was a typo, should be 'MS', of course, but I thought it was funny and fitting enough to leave in. Whadya think?) There's the web site we met through, of course. Do you ever go back to visit, see what's there? Like the frustrated librarian I can be, I keep a list of web addresses which have to do with medicine, MS. disability. Thinking, of course, I will visit sometime. But I haven't so far. How 'boutchu?

You must be a member of the MS Society, US brand, as you have sent me copies of the marvelous newsletters they put out. I really value the Society, with all its weaknesses, for the sense of community it fosters. I can't imagine how lonely it would be to have a very rare disease, so rare there is no one to talk to about it. Our BC Division of MS Canada has recently responded to members' request to offer information on alternative/supplemental medicine and MS. They brought in speakers and broadened our outlook for many of us.

Then there are self-help groups? Have you ever indulged? I did quite some time ago, during my neediest phase. But meetings were not well organized and I thought we all sort of competed for attention, each needing so badly to tell our story. Some groups, I know, are quite informative as well as supportive.

I seem to have very mixed emotions about being with other people with MS. At first, when I used only a cane and got around very well, I felt a bit like a fraud, that I didn't really belong in a group of people in wheelchairs and scooters. Now, when I've attended seminars for PwMS using my scooter, I still want to believe I don't belong there, that this is not really me. I'm still fraudulent because I don't have to use the scooter; I'm still basically a walker. Who knows what complex of emotions is involved in my reaction.

I had to laugh the last time I was at a conference with a lot of other PwMS, many in wheelchairs and scooters. They, like me, were no doubt used to others being quite solicitous and yielding to them, in the washroom or in a lineup. But there we were, with our mobility aids and our weak bladders and no idea of who yields to whom. We had to work out our own traffic rules going in and out of elevators, etc. At one point, I left the scooter outside a room and walked to my seat with my cane to avoid the congestion. En route I saw a woman in a wheelchair who needed someone to push her to her place, so I did. She held my cane for me. And I enjoyed being part of that picture – the blind leading the blind. And I do like being reminded that I am, in some circles, one of the able-bodied; I like being prevented from being petulant or demanding. This being disabled can be addictive if I don't watch myself. I seek, as always, *balance*. I want to pursue my rights as a person with a disability, but not see myself as special in the broad scheme of things.

Where was this going? Community. You see how quickly I turn any topic into a very personal recital. I have reason to worry about losing my balance.

How about you, Julie? Tell me about the US MS Society, whether you attend meetings, etc. Do you feel connected to a community?

A Vancouver joke: A newcomer to Vancouver arrives on a rainy day. She gets up the next day and it's raining. It also rains the day after that, and the day after that. She goes out to lunch and sees a young kid and, out of despair, asks, "Hey, kid, does it ever stop raining around here?" The kid says, "How should I know? I'm only six."

Julie to Linda:

I loved the Vancouver joke. It reminded me of a letter I wrote home to my mother when my husband and I lived in Scotland (he was in the US Navy at the time). A statement that I made to her was that on the day I was writing, it was the 37th straight day of rain. That wasn't kidding either. We had gotten quite used to it, but she never forgot that line, because it sounded so awful to her. It wasn't really. It was a nice gentle rain most of the time, and the environment was so green and beautiful. We just walked around with big umbrellas, and kept the tops up on the baby prams so that they didn't shrink or wrinkle.

Now then, in answer to your questions. Wow, I don't do

any of the things you asked about. I don't belong to news groups. I don't really have many connections in the MS community . . . a couple of friends who have MS and with whom I talk periodically. We compare notes, laugh a little and sometimes cry a little. I am a member of the local and national MS societies, but I usually only take advantage of the publications . . . journals and books from their libraries. Of course, among their literature are numerous donation requests, but I consider them my favorite cause, and readily respond.

There is one thing, however, that I do a lot of. That is to take advantage of the Internet. I have several web sites that I visit frequently: MS Society, Teva-Marion, the manufacturer of Copaxone, IMSSF, MISF, Baylor College of Medicine, MS Crossroads, several medical journals, and some others when I find them. I am a voracious reader of medical info, partly from habit (did it when I was working) and partly from current disease involvement. I do a lot of Internet searching, especially if I have a specific question or have heard about some new and interesting research topic. I'd be happy to share some of my web addresses with you. I don't keep them all on file, but I do the ones that I frequently visit. Just let me know.

As far as self-help groups go, there is one associated with the water exercise group that I used to attend regularly. I say used to because the instructor that is currently involved with the group is bent on endurance training and can be very frustrating to work with, so I haven't been going. The class does meet every other week as a self-help group after the exercise session, however, and when I attend the exercise class, I also attend the self-help group. I often come away feeling frustrated though because it becomes a marathon of trying to top one another's trouble with "mine is worse than yours", and I don't like that. There are periodic teleconferences, which can be attended at various sites, locally or all across the country, presented by the National MS Society. They are also available on the Internet and that's how I usually attend. There is one that has been presented for the past two weeks and will conclude on this coming Saturday. After the last session, it too will be available at the National MS Society web site.

I enjoyed your washroom story. I had a similar experience in a department store when three people, one in wheelchair and two on scooters, descended upon the ladies' room simultaneously. Name the odds of that occurring . . . but it did, and all of us politely laughed, while each individually wanted to run over the other two and exercise their assertiveness. I lucked out. I got second place . . . could have been worse.

Hey, you never did tell me when your birthday is. I know you have one, so I'm waiting. Let me in on it!

Linda to Julie:

I rely on members of the MS newsgroups to distill the bulk of info. out there and feed me what's relevant and reliable. There are members with a very good grasp of medical research protocols, as well as their own personal experience with MS. I generally loose my way at the second or third four-syllable word in a research article, I'm afraid. After a lifetime in school settings, I have a hard time reading for detail unless there's a test on it.

But I keep a list of web sites and do visit occasionally so I would like the addresses of your faves if you can send them easily. There's the frustrated librarian in me – organizing and cataloguing more than using. Tell me more about what you like to get on the Net – to keep up to date with the research? reports from the clinics? personal testimonials?

Aren't we lucky to be dealing with MS in 1999 and not 1969, pre-computer days? People must have been very isolated, especially in smaller places where you might not even have a self-help group. Like people now dealing with rare disorders – a lonely struggle. Whereas I have more potential contacts and sources of information than I can handle. One spin-off of all this, I think, is how well informed PwMS are. One of the neurologists at a seminar here was shocked to realize the knowledge base of many of the audience. It's in our best interest to keep them on their toes and not patronizing us. Ah, the world is a'changing, is it not?

As to my birthday: Now, why on earth would I give you mine when you did not supply yours? (You didn't give it to me before, did you?) I'll show you mine if you show me yours.

Julie to Linda:

My birthday is March 3 by the way. I thought I did tell you, but then it might have been a letter I thought I wrote, but actually didn't. Have you ever done that?

Linda to Julie:

We're both fish! My birthday is March 7, another Pisces. What does that say about us?

Yes, yes, yes, I too sometimes get confused – my thing is not to know if I actually did something or if it was in a dream, or maybe has not even that level of real. I don't think that happened PMS. ("Prior to MS", not the other one.) But maybe it did. I can't remember.

Can I vent a bit here? I had yet another conversation recently of a type which at best, perplexes me and at worst, has me seeing red. It goes like this: I'm talking to a woman who's a senior and she's complaining about her legs and reduced mobility. This neighbor said she was so tired after walking only around a couple blocks. Thinking that putting it into perspective might make her feel not so frustrated, I said, "I wish I could walk that far." At which point, she asks me how old I am. I tell her 52 and she replies, "I'm 78!" in an angry, accusing tone that I took to mean, "But you're young, so it's not so bad for you." Not worth mentioning, except that similar things have happened before. One person told me I would only understand physical difficulty when I reached her age (80). Both these women are very mentally alert, physically quite well. Both obviously having a great deal of trouble with the fact that they're aging. Neither saw the tragic irony in the fact that a much younger person already can do less than they can. On the bright side – as a senior, I'm bound to have more understanding, and be less frustrated with the aging process. That is bright, isn't it?

It's the end of a funny MS week. I had a wonderful, very long day last weekend, when a friend and I drove the Duffy Lake Road, a beautiful drive in the mountains, with lakes and rivers alongside, and no traffic lights or signs for 100km. We were out for twelve hours, I did half the driving, and I felt fine. A short two days later, the weather changed, and a low-pressure system came in. I felt my legs stiffen as the day wore on, and I was hobbling around, not walking. I cancelled an appointment yesterday, went back to bed when I usually do a walk in the park. But I was able to do my tutoring, which was the priority for the day. I drive to the home of the two boys, which gets me out of the apartment. One and a half hours was tiring, but I had enough energy to enjoy it.

Today my legs are still a little reluctant, and my energy not high, but better than the last two days. I'll take it easy, no shopping, no errands today, as I have tickets for a concert tonight. Getting there on my scooter, with the Handidart, (adapted bus) is not a problem, but I want to have enough spirit/energy to enjoy it when I get there. A week ago I had trouble walking, but was otherwise quite capable of enjoying a full day out. Now I can't go to the store and a concert on the same day. It's harder, I think, for friends to cope with this, than me, to understand the contract I have with MS. i.e., I accept that I have to keep some 'money in the bank' if I have plans to take it out later on.

Time for a wee rest before I get ready for the concert. Hope the weather is being kind to you, and you're feeling well.

Julie to Linda:

Hey . . . fellow fish!
You know, I'm married to one also . . . Michael was born on March 8. What does that say about us? I'm not sure! But it could account for why we tend to think a lot alike about many things. Same deranged sense of humor too! Were you able to get into the "Jooley's Joint" web site? That is really a nice service that she provides. What a wonderful way to meet a terrific new friend!!

I do use the research information as leads to new work on the horizon in lots of different categories: clinical trial conclusions particularly pertaining to drug development, research focused on search for cause, etc., etc. I've left my medical job, but haven't lost my thirst for medical information especially since I have such a personal interest in health issues.

Our Memorial Day holiday was Monday, and so because of the nice long weekend, we spent lots of time in the yard. We have a very animal friendly yard (like lots of birds, squirrels, rabbits), and do everything we can to encourage them . . . with food, water, etc. The weather was beautiful, so on Sunday we had the kids and grandkids over for the day. I had no idea how much all five of the little ones like riding on my lap on my scooter. I don't think it (the scooter) has ever had a workout like that. As a matter of fact, I don't remember when I did either.

Your drive along Duffy Lake Road sounded wonderful . . . very relaxing and therapeutic too.

It's terrific that you are able to move around Vancouver by way of the Handidart. Do you have any problems accessing seating in the theater or other places where you enjoy going? How about . . . have you ever taken the scooter to a restaurant or a beauty shop? I can use canes yet in places like that, but it is very difficult if I need to travel any distance from my car. Moving around between display racks in a department store can make me a little cranky, and on numerous occasions, I have complained. Usually, I'm polite about it, but it has pushed my hot button a couple of times, and I've made significant noise about it.

Your "vent" was fun to read because I have definitely had conversations like that. They do sort of tweak a nerve, don't they? And, you wonder how those people would have dealt with MS. I personally would like to try just aging regular like, ya' know?

You know, Linda, I'm very interested in how you deal with MS without the support of immediate family members. There are so many functions of daily living that are impeded. How do you enlist help and from whom? I know that you are a very positive thinking and independent individual, but who provides your emotional support? We all need it sometimes. And, the biggie, how do you manage to keep honoring your contract with MS and all of its resulting routines and obligations? When I start to let things go, such as exercise or social activity, someone gives me a psychological nudge. I sometimes don't even notice that I'm becoming an observer more than a participant, but they do and it doesn't last long. Anyway, how do you deal with those times?

Well, I'm going to sign off here . . . hope you're well, and that the sun is shining in Vancouver.

Linda to Julie:

So we're both fish! What kind do you think you are? I'm definitely a Sucker.

What on earth are we going to do, Julie, when we actually meet in person? I mean, having discovered so much in common, and having communicated so easily with e-mail, what if we are real strangers in person? What if you can't stand me and I dislike you immensely? You'll be gentle . . . won't you? I promise to be kind. I still think the best approach is if we each have a laptop computer available; if face to face proves too uncomfortable, we can retreat and do what's worked well so far – send an e-mail. Take tables at opposite ends of a restaurant or something, and write away.

On to scooter yarns. I too 'cane it' in small shops along the local shopping strip. I take the scooter on a scooter tote at the back of the car when I go to the mall, where I want to go to more than one shop. Department stores are definitely a problem, which I solve by telling people at the cash register (we don't seem to have salespeople available on the floor any more) that I can't maneuver without doing a lot of damage to their racks of little lacey panties and sexy bras. I tell them what I'm looking for and they bring me something to choose from. I am under no illusions here – I'm sure my photo is posted in the staff room with a big warning notice, "Difficult Customer . . . Avoid if possible." When they place racks further apart, I'll do my own shopping. Meanwhile, I don't mind being the one to nudge them along the learning curve. There are shops on the street I can't get into at all with the scooter and I wonder what people do who can't leave their mobility aid outside and 'hoof it'. I find 'accessible' still often means navigable for someone in a wheelchair or scooter, accompanied by a walker of the living, breathing kind.

Nice segue into your questions about coping with MS without close family handy. After days of thinking about your questions and wondering what a truthful answer would be, I must admit my thoughts are still a bit of a jumble. If I just spew forth, maybe you can put the ideas in some kind of order and find some sense?

I can turn most of your questions around. And ask, for example, how on earth you find enough energy, patience, strength to maintain a house and relationships with all your family, and occasionally look after your grandkids. Since I know that's not all you do in life. Mike works full time so he's hardly a househusband. In other words, Julie, I think we all fashion a life to our own tastes, and adapt, as needed, to maintain it. I have a homemaker once a week to keep the place livable. I still drive and carry the scooter on the car so am pretty self-reliant. I live much like any single female. I continue to think that the struggle to do my own shopping is good for me. I do that using the scooter or the car. I have stimulation and challenge, the keys to a good life for me, from tutoring, writing, and keeping on top of this Mystery Show (MS). As for emotional support, I lead a simple life with only a small, demanding dog to look after. I appreciate very much the freedom I have to indulge myself and keep the contract with MS (no high stress, lots of rest, whenever I need it, some daily exercise with the dog). I have enough friends to provide support when needed. I have to be honest and say that I do yearn at times for a sense of community, but that isn't necessarily related to being alone. In fact, a person can be alone even when there are lots of people about.

Vancouver is a big city and I have yet to find my community here. I live in a wonderful neighborhood, but that's different than a community. MS is a factor, in that I don't have the energy to be as gregarious and sociable as I'd like or commit to clubs, etc. But, basically I am a loner and relish the total freedom I have to live life the way I choose. I love being able to collapse when I come home from grocery shopping. But, then, if I weren't alone, I'd have help and wouldn't need to collapse, would I? I think dealing with how someone else is coping with my MS would be very stressful for me. So being alone feels like the right lifestyle, given that MS is itself a constant Mate-Sort of.

I can be organized and efficient because there's little to prevent me from keeping to a routine exercise program, keeping track of the vitamins and supplements I take, keeping track in a journal of my physical ups and downs. I probably couldn't be as good a steward of myself if there were other people to deal with. But then, I wouldn't have to, would I? My life works for me, and is a good one, with lots of quality time. It is not perfect, not without both physical and emotional bumps and ruts, but I wouldn't trade it, MS and all. (That is not to say that, in the dead of night, I don't at times dislike the feeling of being on the edge, of doing this tightrope without a net.)

As for having no partner (you were wondering if I would

touch on that, admit it!), I told a friend some years ago I would love to be married again – but only on Friday nights and Sunday afternoons. Now that would be perfect! If I had a partner, with needs and desires of his own (i.e. not a cardboard cutout), I would need the psychological nudges you mentioned, and would, I'm sure, come to rely on them. I'm able to cope on my own partly because I have no choice, partly because I've adapted to do what I need to now and partly because I'm a selfish egomaniac.

Basically, I believe that our job is to make the most of the cards we are dealt, and it's hard, even futile, to compare your hand to mine. The car driver does not lament the fact that they cannot travel the mountain bicycle paths and cyclists enjoy bicycling even without windshield wipers. (I warned you my thoughts might wander and you might have to piece this together, didn't I?)

Thanks for asking, Julie. I really enjoy learning about how you play your cards, though your hand is so different from mine; I can still learn a trick or two. Maybe you will share with me how MS has affected your relationship with Mike, or how you both have ensured that it doesn't, in any significant way. You see, for me, that appears to be far more difficult for someone with MS than living alone. So – back to you.

Sometimes I wish life would be boring for just a little while – routine, dull. But I think ongoing change is a given for anyone who's getting older and is growing/maturing in the process. Add a chronic, unstable health condition like MS into the equation, and the need to continually adapt to change increases substantially. Sometimes it's difficult to remember life PMS (Prior to MS).

Linda to Julie:

Someone asked me the other day how my life has changed since I found out I have MS? Yikes! I told him I was sure the answer would take a few hours once I had thought it through, and that in itself might take days. Can you help me out here, maybe with a list of categories, all the aspects of life which have changed?

But he did start me thinking. The aspect which I enjoy the most thinking about is just that – my thinking. My whole view of life is different – bigger, wiser, more mature. I have an awareness which I never had before of the life of people who do not fit the comfortable, middle-class mold. And of the whole field of disability, health, medicine, etc. I have a new attitude toward my own health: it sometimes costs money, out of pocket, to maintain it; there's no one to take responsibility for it besides me, so I'd better; my well-being is holistic, more than physical or emotional health alone.

And language. I wrote something last week of "not only people with disabilities but the general public as well". Oh dear me! Is that a Freudian slip? Do I have a hard time accepting People with Disabilities as part of the general public? I became disabled more than ten years ago; my language has obviously not yet caught up. I hope it does not truly reflect my thinking.

In a way my view of disabilities is narrower than it was. I know from my own experience as well as the hundreds of others I have been in contact with, either personally of through reports and stories, that a disability is not a permanent tragedy, that the human spirit is strong and can prevail. That quality of life comes in many forms, from many sources. Most people are visually disabled at some point in their life; few think of wearing glasses as a tragedy, nor having to carry a pair in a case at all times, nor the fact that their glasses are always in the room where they are not. I now see any disability as a huge, very, very huge inconvenience, some bigger than others. Legs are so much more convenient than canes and walkers and wheel-chairs and scooters, no matter how much fun kids think they are. But we still manage to get around, don't we?

And I can pontificate for boring hours on the difference between a disability and a disease. I like to do that from time to time when someone mistakes my use of a scooter with a wheel-chair athlete's. Those guys who play wheelchair basketball are top-notch athletes without self-powered legs. Someone using a wheelchair because of a disease like MS? I don't think so.

How would you answer such a question? Would you even try? How about this question – what is the most significant impact MS (or being disabled) has made on your life?

Julie to Linda:

Just back from a trip. Oh, WOW, it was hot . . . hot . . . hot in Tennessee. And, of course, humid too. It's a good thing I wasn't trying to do anything vigorous. Mike and I did have a nice trip, though, and got in some valuable visiting with some dear, long-time friends. We need to do that every once in a while.

I got to thinking . . . dangerous that is, but I did it anyway. As a result of having MS and the gradual loss of critical func-tions, I seem to be looking at other people with a much different set of expectations. What I mean is this: In years past, I really was not impressed with the manners of the aver-age person on the street. Though I've always liked people in general, I definitely felt that there was a lack of basic courtesy and consideration out there, and that if one was to fall over on the street, most people would keep right on going. Maybe even, they'd step over you if you got in their way.

Well, as this Mighty Stupid disease has advanced, and I have become less than hale and hardy, I'm seeing things I didn't used to. I actually watched as a lady who was trying to get to a door before me so that she could help me, fell on the floor herself. The poor thing. I felt so bad for her. She hit her knees pretty hard as she bolted out of nowhere to assist me. That was for sure above and beyond the call of duty. I truly appreciated her kindness. I'm actually seeing lots of kindness in people these days. I get a lot of offers of aid anytime I'm out. It's sometimes awkward in that someone holding a door to help can, on the contrary, be an obstacle to my passing through it as I require a lot of floor space. But the thought is there, and the spirit is wonderful. I've had people offer to help put my scooter in the van, little kids offer to carry something for me, etc., etc. I think that those people were always out there. I just hadn't taken the time to notice. Actually, I don't think I allowed others to help me very often . . . damn independent cuss, I was. You know, when you slow down, the roses do smell better.

I think that in the past, I had some difficulty in trusting that anyone could take care of my needs any better than I could. I'm a slow learner in this area, I guess. My level of trust along these lines has blossomed considerably, since I require more support in areas I used to handle on my own.

Oh well, it's a shame we start to get smart after 50!

Linda to Julie:

I recently wrote something for the MS Bulletin on Balance; the article has long ago been sent in, but I'm still pondering the topic. How to achieve balance in our lives even though we have a sometimes all-consuming disease. I wrote: It's hard to keep your balance when you have MS, but are still mobile. It's not always easy to walk or step down off a curb. And it's downright treacherous, I've found, to reach up for something in the closet and look around at the same time. But there's another balance that is equally difficult to achieve – the philosophical one – the balance between extremes, the middle ground, the golden mean. And there's no cane to help with that one.

I went on to talk about the balance needed between paying too little and too much attention to the disease. And the balance between under and over-stimulation/challenge.

One of the balances I have to work at which would not be a factor for you, I suppose, is the social one – being around only people with MS, having more and more friends with MS, fewer without.

Lastly, I wrote, "Perhaps the balance I struggle with most is dealing with other people. How to accept well-meant, kind offers of assistance without becoming dependent, or losing my own integrity. How to refuse offers without making the people feel criticized for offering. And how to tell them about living with MS, but not more than they can absorb. How to be honest, without raising their sympathy quotient."

I have no idea if anyone else on this planet relates to any of this, or if I am just blowing in the wind. What do you think? My self-respect does not depend on having company, though, so please be honest. Am I off balance?

TALKING ABOUT SYMPTOMS

MS is unlike any other disease I know in that symp-toms can affect almost any part of the body (not nails or hair, as far as I know now). In fact, MS symptoms are so pervasive, it's easy to forget that a weakness, a pain, tingling in a muscle could be caused by some-thing besides MS – we are still vulnerable to all the other ailments people can get. I figure most of what I have to deal with can be attributed to the 3M company: MS, Menopause, Middle age. Although no two cases of MS are identical, Flora, Julie and I have been able to share a lot of common experiences and ways to deal with various symptoms.

Linda to Flora:

How are you this very wet morning? The sky is so very gray, I just can't imagine that there is any end to it, that somewhere the sun does shine.

One of the things that has bugged me for a long time in the 'official' talk about MS, I mean what the doctors and researchers and even MS Society talk about almost exclusively is mobility problems. And in my books, that's only a part of the problem, not a small part, but certainly not the whole story. How often do you find an article on cognitive and emotional effects? And in my books, it's the intellectual function, which is the most precious. So, just for fun I have put together a list of all the ways I think MS may have affected my thinking and my emotions; some of these may, I know, be simply an effect of having any chronic disease, not MS in particular. And some, I do hate to admit, may be a function of aging. And some are because my body is now in menopause. I know, I know, there's a lot more happening in my body than just MS. But I have found enough articles on it to confirm many of my suspicions. I wonder what you think. How many of these can you relate to?

Mental fatigue

In the middle of something – a conversation, reading, writing, even a TV show – my brain quits on me. I guess that in itself is not unusual, but this happens to me so quickly – a couple hours of mental effort or less if it's intense. And I don't feel it gearing down; it just stops cold. Aging? Menopause? MS?

Mental confusion

I have a much harder time figuring out the simplest of things – the change owed me when I pay for something, following the plot of a murder mystery, particularly the good British ones, a new card or board game – these I seldom even attempt any more, just too tough. This is most troublesome when I try to learn something new – new program on the computer, etc. My, oh my, that does take me a long time, and I feel like a kid at school again, one of the crows not the bluebirds, as two levels of readers were identified in my Grade one class. Aren't I too young to say this is due to my age? Please, Flora, tell me I'm not that old!

Linear thinking

I think well when I need to deal with only two factors – x as the cause of y. Bob is married to Sue. The earth circles the sun. So far, so good. But please don't confuse me by talking about a sub-topic, like something which affects X, Sue's sister's son ("Who is he again?"), the moon in relation to the earth at different times. (I need to picture it in my mind to keep clear all the orbs moving around in the sky.)

Short term memory

This is one of the MS effects that is often mentioned, the decline in short term memory. This is now much better than it was a few years back, when I couldn't remember all of the seven digits of a phone number if I wanted to keep it in mind until I got to a pen and paper to write it down. I notice something else in connection with it, that short term memory very quickly goes into long term. So if I do remember something, I lose the sense of when it happened. Things I did yesterday I will remember as having happened much longer ago than that, maybe even a week. I have learned to stop saying to people, "So good to hear from you, haven't talked to you in a long time," as they invariably remind me we talked just last week. In my mind it seems like weeks. And weeks seem like months. Remembering names is the most embarrassing place I trip up with short-term memory, I find. I can be introduced to someone and a minute later have forgotten their name. Sometimes this happens even if I make a conscious effort to hold the name in my mind – when another thought pushes it out in the interval.

Word loss

This again is something often mentioned, the inability to remember even easy, common words in the heat of the moment. It's embarrassing if you stop mid-sentence because you can't think of 'cushion' or 'manager.' I find I'm getting good at quick substitution – 'pillow' or 'boss' are close enough. And if I can relax, stop searching for the word in my brain's files, my subconscious will quietly do its thing and give me the word some time later. The same often goes for names I've forgotten.

Names

I have as much trouble confusing names as I do forgetting them. Trying to keep straight two men I worked with, Len and Des. Those names are just too similar, one syllable with an 'e' in the middle. Even after years, I had trouble putting the right name to the right person. I have trouble keeping Michelle and Rachel straight, and again, have to really concentrate to put the right name to the right person.

Fatigue with social intercourse

I never would have thought of conversation as tiring, but it sure is now: in a group, at a meeting, on the phone. An hour is about all I can handle before my inner self is crying, "Please, please, can we just get away from all this racket, maybe go lie down in a corner somewhere?" I like solitude an awful lot more than I ever did before; I used to be rather gregarious, in fact.

Social clumsiness, loss of filters, inhibitions

My pattern of social interaction seems to have changed. My conversation is very direct, with little of the niceties we usually start and end with. I can feel my mind grappling with the point I want to make, the question I want to ask, and not being able to also come up with a social filler or bridge. "Hi, how are you, when is the meeting?" "Good day, can I borrow your big frying pan?" I also cannot filter out things before they leave my mouth and say very inappropriate things sometimes. Making jokes where I shouldn't. I'm an adolescent all over again.

I have absolutely no social graces on the phone. I called a friend this morning and was surprised when her husband answered. So surprised I didn't even say hello to him, just asked directly for her. And I can feel the tension in my mind as it has to adjust from what it expected, and cannot quickly find the appropriate thing to say. More tension, perhaps, because I don't know him all that well although I do not feel uncomfortable with him.

All of this, like my walking, is worse when I'm tired, of course. Which means I don't do anything, physical or mental, for very long before I stop and rest. I find my active, alert day ends about nine p.m. after which I turn on the TV and hope there's a good, but not too esoteric, comedy on to watch.

The very fact that I want to get all this down, make a list, is a reflection of how important it is to me. I take Lethicin, which is supposed to help with memory, and I think the acupuncture helps keep me as 'bright' as I can be (but not brighter than prior to MS, unfortunately). How about you?

Flora to Linda:

Clearly this is an important issue for those folks who are mentally active and therefore aware when they are out of step or have missed a step entirely. How would I manage if I were still at work? Probably fine, except for the current optic neuritis and occasionally getting too tired, because I am pretty skilled at covering my tracks. An example is inventing new ideas (hopefully not new words) in mid-sentence particularly if speaking publicly or at least to a group.

Thinking back, I remember interviewing for a staff position and losing it. What was I saying? (And this was well before diagnosis.) And my co-interviewer didn't help when she said, "You lost it didn't you?" She was right, but she could have covered for me at least for the sake of the confused interviewee! No one's fault but my own but one of those times when you think you are going mad. I learned to keep notes, pay close attention, have a backup question on hand, etc.

Like my friends, some older, some not, I now have more trouble with names. Then other times I find myself recalling addresses, phone numbers, and details of what I thought in the middle of the night. Was life always this unpredictable? Is everybody's on occasion? Garbling syllables and vowels does happen at times, and you are right, more often at the end of the day.

Fatigue with social intercourse is nicely put. "Why don't they go away?" You by the way are too young to claim old age and general crotchitiness.

To be specific, I don't get hit by mental fatigue in the same way you describe. Certainly I can't keep up real effort for long, so I space bits of the day and do letters or business in the morning for example. As for mental confusion, this I get as a panic response with high emotional content if for example I am on the phone and get asked for what I cannot quickly provide such as care card number. It's an eyesight problem combined with tremors preventing me from quickly flipping through my addresses/info that I do keep on hand. And if there is a heavy-duty emotional component, like a discussion with our accountant, I can be sent into shakes and really can't go on with a discussion, never mind make decisions. Needless to say, taking notes that I cannot later decipher is impossible. So I phone him/her back when I've had a chance to calm down and think. Does this sound familiar?

And I retract what I said about doing well at work. Thinking fast and under stress isn't really possible too often. Word loss certainly happens, but as I've said, I'm good at covering. Your loss of filters comment I don't think is a big one for me, I have had a number of conversations with friends when I am aware of carrying a counselor-like role that I think have been OK. Re: poor memory of movies and TV. I count on this. So many TV shows are repeats the good ones sometimes are worth watching again, particularly when I have no idea "who did it".

As for resting, I need it if I haven't had enough sleep. An hour down, with feet up, not sleeping but with eyes closed keeps me able to get through the rest of the day and evening. As for medication, I have started Gingko Biloba daily but have no idea what or whether it helps. And age may be a factor for us but not much. Whatever we intend to do and do manage we have to keep better organized than other folks. And we need a little help from our friends or at least I certainly do.

Flora and I also agree on the benefit of counselling, the need for psychological wellness.

Flora to Linda:

I have appreciated your comments on cognitive factors that influence your life. And in looking at them, I realize that they are without exception the sort of factor/problem/issue I deal with by what I loosely interpret as counselling. It's my method of looking for explanation and ideas for coping. "Tell me why this is happening? What can I do about it?" Definitely not limited to a session in a social worker's office or a polite way of referring to visits to a psychiatrist. Not that I would discount either of them.

For me, counselling covers a lot of general territory. I have had good advice and referral as well as treatment from an acupuncturist. I have seen a behaviour science counselor for in depth discussion and exploration by going way back in my life. Hands-on treatment and helpful therapy as well as new ideas and practical help from a pranic healer and cranial sacral therapist.

My family doctor is also a counselor and explores emotional reactions and personal problems with me. There are all sorts of perspectives on a disease and coping with a disease and its effects. Part of my helping group as I define them (some professional, some not, some downright far-out) are not in touch with each other at least not regularly and not about me. Do I sound like a help junkie? And this from a professional social worker who admirably practiced more social planning, management, and even research than proper social work. And I have more to explore; Yoga has been helpful as exercise and sleep skills but I will do more to learn meditation. You made a comment recently that fit my exploring mode. You mentioned the subconscious, a heightened ability. Can you say more about this? I know for me it ties to the mind-body-emotions connection we have heard so much about. But strategies for tapping in to that particular part of brain activity? Sounds rather wonderful.

Linda to Flora:

I don't remember what I said about the sub-conscious (are you surprised?) but I can talk anytime about anything at the drop of a word, so here goes. I think counselling has helped me get in touch with parts of myself which were pretty shy before. I recognize my sub-conscious as a valid and useful part of me, so I give it jobs to do. "I'm going to sleep/rest now, but I want you to work on finding that word while I do." I dream more too, but I'm sorry to say my dreams are just as boring as they ever were – just documentaries, a little revisionist history of my life. Last night, for instance, I dreamt I was still working as an educational consultant, giving a workshop. Some of the people in the dream were those I worked with twenty-five years ago. But there was nothing in my dream to take to anyone for interpretation. How jealous I am of people who dream weird and wonderful fantasies, with mythical creatures and science fiction scripts! Maybe I'll ask my sub-conscious to come up with one like that for my amusement!

As for counselling, I've seen several counsellors in the past and a couple of psychiatrists when I couldn't afford counsellors. I used the employee assistance plan at work which provided confidential counselling through an outside agency when I felt really stressed-out trying to deal with MS and work. I eventually found my own solution to that one, when I went on Long Term Disability. And I did quite a bit on my own (i.e. paid for myself) when I first started having serious trouble, after 1987. I think I can deal with the MS better if I am otherwise very healthy, and that means emotionally as well as physically. I can't afford any longer the luxury of demons, those little gremlins in my psyche which drag me down, like the perfectionist nature I have had most of my life, hindrances to healthy personal relations, etc. I don't think I'm particularly troubled; it's just that I am affected physically by any emotional imbalance, so I have to look after it.

In that way, I feel I've benefited from MS. It has made me examine and rethink myself. I just recently felt strong enough to once again embark on the journey of self-discovery and have gone back into counseling; I find friends are too kind to really help me examine things, and quite often they cannot look at me objectively. I really appreciate a skilled outsider who can pose questions and help me learn new strategies. I agree that the mind-body link is strong; I've done a lot for my body for years (acupuncture, mostly), and realized that I had more or less ignored the mind part of the equation. I feel quite privileged to be able to indulge in the exercise and have known for a long, long time that I could not take my health for granted as I once did, that it is going to require more than average amounts of time, concentration and money. Also that I have very little in the way of options. Thanks for raising the topic, Flora. I'm very interested in it, and think it's one of the many areas where we're left to our own devices, for the most part.

Then there are the symptoms I've never heard of, physical changes I'm not sure I would attribute to MS. Like the change in my voice.

Linda to Julie:

Have you ever heard anyone mention a Voice Clinic at your hospital? I heard of it only through chatting with someone who knew nothing of MS; I was simply mentioning my frustration with what I perceived as a weakness in my voice, (can you believe I have trouble talking?) and my loss of the ability to sing. We're not talking operatic levels here, of course, only the ability to join in when sing-fests erupt. I used to love to sing, and miss the ability to entertain myself, if nothing else. Of course, if they could give me the voice of a Bartoli or Norman, I wouldn't complain! I have trouble projecting, which is most apparent on the phone, which is very exhausting as it takes a lot of energy and concentration to be clear and loud enough to articulate well and be heard. At times I have sort of lost my voice as you might after running uphill (Did we ever run uphill? Why on earth?). I was happy to know there was someone who could check out my vocal machinery, someone I could talk to about what was happening. I got an appointment by phoning the ENT clinic in the hospital, sending in an info. sheet and getting a doctor's referral.

I met with two doctors and a speech therapist. With a camera in my throat taping my very sexy vocal cords as they undulated in and out; I vocalized and watched on a screen. And for the first time, I saw me talking, while a microphone monitored my every squeak. The experts had me do a number of exercises, as well as just talk to them. Their conclusion? Definite weakness in the vocal cords, worse on the left (surprise! – my weak side). What can they offer? A workbook and an eight-week course on vocalizing to help teach techniques, the sort of thing which professional singers use. I bought the book and will try to go through the exercises; I think the vocal cords are like legs, in that I need to put them through a range-of-motion pattern of exercises.

This was one of the more pleasant medical encounters I have had dealing with MS on this side of the ocean. I would highly recommend it to anyone troubled by changes in their voice.

That's it – more than you ever wanted or needed to know about the voice clinic and my vocal cords. Have you ever noticed any weakness like this? Let's start a contest "Weirdest MS Symptom". No rules, just throw anything in the hopper you can find a way to connect to MS, I know you're good at that.

Julie to Linda:

I have never experienced anything like you describe, and I don't know of one in this area. It sounds wonderful. My voice has not changed with MS, at least I'm not aware of any change. It seems natural that vocal cords and movement of the diaphragm would be affected, and I wonder why there is not more attention paid to the issue, especially with the number of MS centres there are available in all countries. It's a question I'll ask my neurologist the next time I see him. That won't be for a while, though.

And from Flora on the same topic:

I think my voice is pretty well as was, although I no longer can sing. I used to sing a lot, particularly to the children. My current effort is to find a CD or two with words I can sing along with – Mozart doesn't do it. Ella Fitzgerald doesn't either. Maybe I need some Bing Crosbie or Gene Autry. More like a choice my parents would make, however. Or grownup stuff I sang when I was a little kid! The exercises can make a huge difference over time. Certainly voice is a loss you don't need and especially if it's recoverable.

Canadians love to talk about the weather – we have so much of it. Canadians with MS have more reason to talk about it, as it affects us dramatically at times. Before doctors had the MRI (Magnetic Resonance Imaging) one of the tests leading to diagnosis was often the results of a long, hot bath – did the person suffer the common MS symptom of extreme fatigue?

Linda to Flora:

How are you doing? More precisely, how were you doing yesterday? Did you find any air worth breathing? any life worth living? anything worth doing?

I don't think I've ever suffered so much from the heat. It's not the temperature itself that gets me; it's that muggy air, the humidity. I was sitting out at a neighbour's place in the morning, and suddenly The Fatigue just descended on me like a wave. I wasn't doing anything physical at the time, just chatting. My mind ground to a quiet, insidious halt, such that it took a great deal of effort to put words to anything. For the rest of the day, I alternated between activity and bedrest, in about equal portions. Which led to worry and depression, in about equal portions. I can usually talk myself out of that, but it takes time. The heat alone doesn't do this to me, but I feel positively oxygen-deprived on muggy days. How about you? Hope you're breathing and living well.

Fatigue is the least understood and perhaps the most frequent symptom I have to deal with. Sometimes my mind and body are in total harmony, close to comatose. Not really an exacerbation, it's just a few days of real weakness and fatigue. And it's so nice to have friends to vent with about it.

Linda to Flora:

I'm writing to you not because I have anything interesting or illuminating to say but because I'm too flat to do anything else. MS flat. Fatigued. Spiritless. Ass dragging. You don't have this, do you? Can I tell you about it . . . please.

I was in good form all last week, spirit and drive, physical and mental energy. I walked more and was determined that I would soon be walking right around the park. I worked on TB (The Book), phoned you, had ideas, felt alive. Then on Monday I woke up feeling . . . different. I hadn't had a good sleep, and had been up with the dog a couple of nights, so didn't take it too seriously. (Not good, by the way, means eight or nine hours, instead of ten or eleven.) I did my volunteer work at the MS Society, which was even more hectic than usual, but still I managed and got home in one piece. Not feeling, however, up to a meeting I had planned to go to. On Tuesday, I went to an appointment to check out a Qi Gong practitioner, which was awful. His office was a real zoo, and I left, after waiting for forty-five minutes. Was that stressful? I guess maybe. It certainly wasn't fun or pleasant. After that. I felt worse but went ahead with a plan to have dinner with a friend, which may have been a big mistake. I had a very inconvenient bowel incident after dinner, which in itself was quite stressful. Wednesday I felt worse and today the same. This morning my homemaker cleaned up the place while I kept popping back into bed for twenty minutes or so. I went through the motions of sorting out some stuff with her help, but felt neither interest in doing it nor satisfaction in getting it done. Just dragging through what I felt I had to do. I slept for two solid hours after lunch, took Sashi to the park, but did no walking, and here I am. I've been taking the same supplements and vitamins as usual, even took extra Royal Jelly. But still I'm flagged. Why? Where did I go wrong – too much activity last week? Too much stress this week? Too little exercise this week? Too much last week? Hormones? Food? How long will this last? And what should I do to speed a return to some vitality? MS – the Mystery Show. For me this kind of fatigue is the worst symptom I have to deal with. How about you?

Later: On reading this over, and thinking back over this week, I realize just how many stressful experiences there were. My poor fragile body cannot handle stress, I know. It's all a little clearer now. Thanks for being there for me to write at.

Flora to Linda:

It is indeed a mystery disease. My rule of thumb is that everything will take vastly longer than expected. A bit like the rule that says if anything can go wrong, it will. But underneath it all, I am an optimistic person – even flagrantly optimistic. My take is that even after the down days, and some can be really dreadful, it's all part of the learning mode I seem to have to talk about. Though I have to accept that no matter how well or how quickly I learn, I'm not necessarily going to win or change the rather strange rules of play. So keep your chin up.

On the other hand, I have been lucky not to suffer particularly from fatigue. Not that I push my luck by spending two days in a row without a good rest or the chance to sit for a couple of hours. But the dreadful, debilitating tiredness that others feel has not, as yet, been my lot.

Linda to Flora:

Have you never felt the fatigue, which is the hallmark of MS for so many people? Even during a relapse? I'd say you're lucky, but it is more honest to say, I think, that there is enough cosmic sense in the world not to take away the strength you need to deal with vision and mobility problems.

Since you don't suffer from fatigue (grr!) I guess you wouldn't have experienced "The Metamorphosis". Slowly becoming someone different, with no script for the new role your body is assigning. Here's how it goes, with today's experience fresh in my mind. You did say you were dying to know the details, didn't you?

I had arranged to meet four others (staff) from the MS Society for Dim Sum at ten a.m. I don't as a rule go out in the morning, and there was just a bit of pressure to get ready by then; I got up at eight, spent a little more time than usual in the bathroom dealing with bowels that do not like to be rushed. But I got cleaned up and felt good. Luckily I knew where the restaurant was so there was no stress getting there; I arrived quite calm and feeling ready to engage in conversation, and eat, of course. We had a nice time, with easy conversation, laughs, and no food fights. But by 11, I could feel my mental engine starting to sputter; I looked at my watch in disbelief – I'd only been out for an hour (but I had been up and active for three). I withdrew just a little from the conversation, but was still able to throw something in now and again.

But I was aware of the metamorphosis, the change from participant to observer. The slight, but growing desire on my part to just sit in quiet peace, with no talking. I enjoyed myself, in spite of this, for another half-hour or so. But then, the MS in me was quite loud; meanwhile, the social me was eager to carry on. There was an inner tussle, and finally I felt so uncomfortable I just had to leave; I had no drive, no mental energy to cope with the socializing, and became Linda the recluse, trying, but feebly, to engage in parting niceties. I watched the other four with their energy not yet on the wane, it was only mid-day!, and I felt both insulted by my MS and eager to get away from people who made comparison hard to avoid. I'm sure they saw little of my metamorphosis, but in my mind it was all too obvious, painful and awkward. I had once again become someone I am not used to being. I'm much more comfortable being the gregarious one who dominates the conversation than the retiring type. The world at large may not, I realize, be sorry for this change in me.

That's my MS news to date. Next challenge coming up: I have agreed to drive a couple girls to their prom tonight. Others will drive up in limousines; these two will arrive in a car with a scooter tote and a handicap placard. I ask others to treat me no differently, so what's the problem in my head? I have to get around the idea of feeling a little sorry for the girls and wishing our style was going to be more cool than coping – for their sake, of course. But let me be rational about this . . . I am going to be OK with it all . . . really . . . I'm sure.

One thing the MS does not mess with is enjoying the excitement of my neighbour's daughter as she shows me her gown, the shoes, her graduation photo. That's the best part of the whole thing for me, and it is totally unblemished by MS.

Can you relate to any of this? It's always good to write it down and give these feelings a voice. Thank you for listening.

Linda L. Ironside

_____

Flora to Linda:

I've been thinking about your comments on fatigue. There is a definition problem throughout the MS community not aided by neurologist et al. Is fatigue daily, occasional but all embracing? Certainly it's very personal.

For me it does not happen every day or the same time of day. I feel dozy some days, take a sit-up nap and then feel like getting on with something. However I knew from my most severe exacerbation 18 months ago that working at the pace I did in the past was not possible. Occasionally, I go to bed and seep soundly for two hours without affecting my usual night's sleep. But, mostly, I avoid such naps as destructive of regular sleep patterns and managing eight or even nine hours. Regularity is boring and predictable, but it works. But daylong fatigue? No.

Was reminded today however, not to push things. I went downstairs to the basement to search for a range of potting materials for spring. Got them to the stairs and couldn't manage to walk up the stairs all the way. I had to use the sit-down technique and the pots are still sitting at the top of the stairs. Next time, I will have a helper. I will get myself down there and back up too but I will give directions on finding the pots and containers, sit down all the while and be very thankful for willing helpers. For me, this qualifies more as tiredness than fatigue. What do you think? This must be the world's most qualified disorder. Everything "depends".

Linda to Flora:

One of the symptoms I get is an overwhelming sense of weakness in my legs, which I remember feeling prior to MS at the end of a very long hike, especially climbing. I had to basically talk my legs into moving, the instinct to walk was not enough. Bliss was being able to sit down. No pain, no stiffness, just very, very weak. My balance is never very good and when I'm, tired it's worse, of course; I do more wall walking, balancing by touching the walls, left and right. This seems to spread to a big case of general fatigue, where I lose interest in doing much of anything, sitting or standing. My mind gets foggy, my spirit dull. So my legs seem to call the shots; that's where I have to save energy as much as I can. That's where my MS manifests itself the most.

Later, after giving my legs the rest they required, I wrote:

My legs have responded very nicely, but life keeps making more demands. I was feeling rather well, then got a new roommate, a small black hairy one who is absolutely irresistible. Winnie has energy to burn and draws me into all manner of games; then there are the people visiting to meet her. Trips to the vet and the pet food supply. Walks (scooter rides for me) in the park. All of which I used to do with Sashi, but had gotten out of the habit. So my body is once again complaining, although I sure sleep well, total exhaustion does that! But this is OK; I know what it is and that I will soon find my equilibrium again, as Winnie becomes less of a novelty and more independent. I am looking forward to an extended period of time with no new challenges and not too much stimulation. (I sure sound old, don't I?)

Linda L. Ironside

The topic of exercise, like many others, is a difficult one to get a clear picture of – how much is needed to slow down atrophy; how much is too much, leading to muscle fatigue and maybe a worsening of symptoms? I seem to go back and forth on this one, and have erred on both sides, doing too little as well as too much.

Linda to Flora:

A year and a half ago, I was concerned that I was walking less and less, and that my leg muscles might be atrophying more than necessary. So I checked out one of the passive exercisers, and borrowed one (Ex N' Flex) for a week from a very friendly and understanding distributor here in Vancouver. Well, I thought this was just the thing for me, so easy to do while I watched a bit of TV. And I had enough strength in my legs to add a bit of resistance, so I'd be working the muscles. Oops – big oops! How could I have forgotten after nineteen years that MS is a problem of the nerves, that it's the nerves I must pay attention to? But I didn't; I went full steam ahead, twenty minutes twice a day, and felt very righteous about it. I didn't hear my poor nerves calling, "Stop, stop, please stop, we're having trouble here keeping up!" until almost a week of this, when my whole body said, "Tried to warn you, but you like to learn the hard way; we're on strike as of now!" All systems shut down and I was in worse shape for a couple weeks than I'd been for years. This is bad enough, but it was not the first time I'd been so silly. Once before, a trainer in the weight room at the community centre and I both got so excited about my progress that we upped the ante and pushed my nerves to meltdown.

Maybe my experience can serve as a warning to others who might be just a tad too keen.

> MS *is never boring. Or, to put it another way, just when you think you are coping quite well with all the symptoms you have, up pops another one. I wasn't really bored with the same 'ol, same 'ol (fatigue, mobility, balance, bladder, bowels, nystagmus (movement of the eyeball), hand flexibility, cognitive deficits), though, when I suddenly had something else to think about. As always I drew comfort from describing it for Flora.*

Linda to Flora:

I've had a fair bit of vertigo the last few days, which has convinced me to do less with my mind as well as my body for a little while. I don't really notice anything unusual until I'm sitting on the bed and flop back to lie down. Then – Ooooh! My head is in the spin cycle; I feel my brains sloshing around and it doesn't stop for a few seconds. Not exactly painful, even a little interesting, but once is enough. It's very much like being on one of the rides at the fair when you're a kid. You scream like crazy, but you'll do it again, because there's something in it that's fun? The feeling of being on the edge? Which is OK when you know it will stop and you can get off. But when your head goes on this ride all on its own, it is a bit different. And it leaves me with a hangover – a headache and a feeling of pressure that lasts for hours. But I can get off this ride too, just don't move my head too quickly.

Linda L. Ironside

I've taken a couple nasty falls in the past when I raised my arms high at the same time that I moved my head – someone said we shouldn't move our head in two planes at once, which clarifies the situation for me.

Now, if I can just remember that when I bend over to pick up something, I must come up again very slowly or when putting something on the top shelf, not to turn or twist.

It's all interesting, because the human brain is fascinating. Is it ironic or logical that a cerebral person like me has had so much trouble in the head, starting long before MS with that nasty bit of intercranial hypertension back in the 1970s. I wish I'd been alert enough to follow that.

POPPING PILLS, ETC.

In 1996 there was at long last exciting news from the lab for people with MS. The so-called ABC (and R in Canada) drugs were found to help some people in reducing the number or severity of exacerbations. The excitement was understandable, since this was the very first time any drug was found to alter the course of the disease. The drugs are Avonex, Betaseron, Rebif, and Copaxone, the only one which is not a beta interferon. When you mention drugs for MS (or any other disease, I expect), two things send a chill down the spine: side effects and cost.

My medical coverage, through the BC government medical plan and my extended health coverage from my Long Term Disability benefit, is quite extensive. But even the deductibles for some drugs can be too high for many people, especially those on the new drug treatments, which cost in the thousands. So – the stress about the cost of a drug which is supposed to be a help may be a factor in a picture of declining wellness. I was curious to know about Julie's coverage in the US.

Linda to Julie:

We've talked about a lot, you and I . . . you've told me about your body and you've told me about your husband. But . . . well . . . we've never . . . you know . . . talked turkey . . . Dare we now?

No, Julie, I don't think we should drag skeletons out of the closet. And I really don't think we need to divulge our religious convictions, or sexual fantasies. But I am, I have to admit it, keenly interested in your politics. Well, not yours exactly, more your country's. No, that's not even it – what I want to know is the situation with medical coverage for you and others with MS. There, that's not so sensitive, is it?

Here's the dope on this side: medical coverage is the mandate of the provinces, so there's a lot of variance in the country. But every province has a government medical plan, which covers the basics: doctor visits, referrals to specialists, hospital stays. Here in BC I also get twelve visits a year to a certified masseur, or chiropractor. Drugs are covered over the yearly deductible of $800.

Most employees have extended health benefits as part of their contract, which picks up user fees, equipment and supplies (syringes, catheters, bath chair, scooter, walker, etc.), and orthotics. Acupuncture, though recognized, is still not covered by the government. My insurance company will cover it if done by a physiotherapist (like covering my dental work if done by a hairdresser?). They do cover, to a maximum of $275 per year (for each) speech therapists, osteopath, podiatrist, naturopath and psychologist

My Long-Term Disability (LTD) benefit, together with the government disability pension gives me 80% of my salary, to a maximum of $20,000 a year. Until I reach 65. That's when developing an appetite for pet food is going to come in handy, as I will have only a tiny pension from work and the government disability pension.

Apparently in terms of the ABCR drugs, only Betaseron is now covered in BC though a couple other provinces are already covering two or three of them. But even at 80% coverage, there are people who cannot afford it. People without extended health benefits. I don't know how they manage. The MS Society can help a little bit, and is very good at providing equipment.

Ay yai yai, so many figures! I shoulda been an accountant! (Too late to marry one, you think?)

Can you fill me in as to the situation for Americans with MS? Or at least for one American.

Julie:

The politics of health care in the US is certainly different from what you encounter.

Here, the medical coverage is primarily private, and for a great percentage of the population, it is considered a benefit of employment. Most larger employers (like fifty or more people) offer some form of health insurance to people working there. In most of these cases, there is a partial pay clause for the employee (like $50 or so/month) to buy that coverage. When I no longer worked, I lost my full coverage medical insurance (it was really a good policy), and was very concerned about it. Although I had to pay out of my own pocket for devices like my scooter, wheelchair and walker, all of my meds and everything else was paid for at 100%. As the cost of medical supplies and meds here are often not covered, I knew that I would be paying for more myself when I switched to using Mike's employer paid coverage. It's a different policy, underwritten by the John Hancock Life Insurance Co. Mine was called DMC care and it was a self-funded policy with care provided by the medical system I worked for, the Detroit Medical Center.

Anyway, to shorten the description of a very complex and varied system, not all insurers are the same. The policy that Mike's employer provides now is actually very good. I pay approximately 20% of most things and if (or I should say when in our case) we reach $1200 of "out-of-pocket" expenses, they generally cover 100%.

Since September, they've decided to pay for 100% of my Copaxone all of the time, regardless of what my out-of-pocket limit is. That was wonderful news, because last year, I paid $192/month for it plus 20% of all of my other medications.

I do receive some income from the government due to my disability, and after being on these Social Security payments for 24 months, I became eligible for Medicare. This is a government paid (funded by tax dollars) medical insurance which, until I am 65 years old, is my secondary insurer. In other words, they sometimes pay some of the unpaid 20% when my primary insurer has already been billed. When Michael no longer is employed at his current job, we will have no private insurance. I will have Medicare only (that's not nearly the kind of coverage that you enjoy). In no way is massage therapy or home help or anything like that paid.

I just purchased a long-term care insurance policy for Mike, so that if he were ever to become incapacitated, I would be able to afford help with his care. The same company rejected me because of the likelihood that I will need care someday. That's frustrating, but reality.

Acupuncture here, is covered now by a lot of insurers, but only if considered a recognized treatment for the diagnosis involved. MS is usually not. I received full reimbursement for my forearm crutches a few months ago, cause they keep me on my feet, I guess.

It is a complicated system, and one that requires a lot of management on the part of the individual. It pays to be assertive and to keep looking out for oneself. It keeps the brain cells active for sure. I too feel sorry for people who don't have adequate coverage. Some people here, too, receive assistance from the MS Society, and like in Canada, they're very good, I understand, with equipment acquisition.

So we decide to spend the money and get the drugs, conventional or alternative. How will we know if they're working? We react to so many things: our personal psychology, social interactions, hormones, diet, weather – as well as the pills or injections we may be taking.

Linda to Julie:

How on earth can I ascertain if a new treatment is helping or not?

I get acupuncture most weeks, a B12 shot most weeks. A full massage once a month. I occasionally do the moxibustion (TCM form of heat stimulation) on my head. Recently I have been using Progesterone cream or suppository. And a new line of vitamins and minerals (more potent than the drugstore variety?) as well as flavonols (high-powered anti-oxidant?) from Usana (have you heard of them?). I am doing very well right now, much better (bladder, concentration, fatigue), than I was just a few weeks ago, when my legs were so weak it was scary. I would like to continue to do whatever is making the difference. (Weather is ruled out, as I have been feeling better through hot or cold, high or low pressure.) I think it's the bioflavonols, given when I started taking them and when I started feeling better, and not just because the name sounds impressive. But it's hardly a scientific study. And they're expensive. I wish I had your head for science, and a little patience to keep track of all the possible factors in a daily log of wellness.

When I think of how much better I am, even given my recalcitrant legs, than I was a few years ago, I am really thrilled. Not having the stress of work helps a lot! But I'm not stable for long; when I'm in a less well period, or when others (at least two) give a glowing testimonial, I am encouraged to try something new. And, of course, there's an immediate positive effect, accounted for, I think, by the mental boost and renewed hope from anything new. I've learned to wait a month or two before coming to any conclusions.

Julie to Linda:

At any given time I must say, there are quite a few things that alter or account for the way I feel. Like you, I know that hormones and their balance or imbalance have a say in what I'm capable of dealing with. But then so do other major factors over which I have no control, like weather, as you stated, and general conditions of the people around me. I think my response to things like family members' needs, my doctors appointments and other stuff, and obligations that I place on myself like work when I'm doing some & social commitments are probably potentially more stressful because

I have a tendency to let them pile up. By that I mean, I'll have a few good days when I start to feel I can do more than I really can, and then I make promises to myself to do things. I guess it's kind of the old striving to make things like they used to be. Well, usually I don't go off too crazy, but sometimes I get a little carried away, and then I pay with a couple of days when I am virtually worthless. I use worthless in the sense that absolutely NOTHING gets done . . . even the most basic things like cooking supper (we resort to leftover surprises from the freezer). I'm so glad that Mike is so easy to feed. Anyway, I think that my desire to still be all the things I used to be serves to remind me that those things I used to be don't have a place in the current scheme of things. I'm quite happy with the new ways, but I just have to remember what the necessary adjustments are and then I have to remember to apply them. I take more time to rest, using wheels instead of trying so hard to be eye-to-eye with people and stop to smell the roses much more frequently than I used to do.

It all boils down to enabling myself to enjoy myself, and to eliminating the actions or behaviors that get in the way of doing that. Know what I mean? I figure that a person can't control the fact that they have something like MS that causes limitations, but they sure can control how to deal with it. If I'm going to feel worthwhile, I need anything I can get my hands on to enable that. That does require the pursuit of the right mix of medications and trying very hard to eat right (someday I'll get better at that), exercise (I'm so bad at staying regular with it), and then like you other things such as vitamins. I'm not doing anything too terribly fancy with vitamins though. I take a multi-vitamin tablet every day and a calcium supplement. I just figure I probably miss something in my diet and should make up for it with a pill or two.

Linda L. Ironside

I like "Mighty Scrambled." That sure defines us nicely. I haven't been able to think of too many MSisms lately. Maybe by the end of this letter, something will come to mind. I'm going to stop for a while and go to the butcher. We need some food here today. My talk above about freezer surprises prompted me to go look for some. WOW – nothing! I definitely need to go stock up.

Till later,

your (M)ichigan (S)ister

Now most people in Canada have at least some of the new drugs available, though not all are covered by provincial health plans or private insurance (as extended health coverage). Since that time there has been some refinement, a widening of criteria of who might benefit. Both Flora and Julie are on this drug program; their experience confirms what many others have reported – reactions are very individual, and finding the right drug for you is a trial and error process.

Flora to Linda:

Hi! So, my start date is fast approaching. The drug, Betaseron, has been covered by BC medical since last spring. Obviously I am one of the eligible who did not jump at the chance. I was hoping that I would have a good reaction to diet revision but that was not notably the case. I will stay with some of those diet decisions and some of the supplements as well as the energy work, which simply helps me feel better.

My progression over the past two years since I stopped work is evident. Two years ago I managed well on a cane. Now I need a walker and, on long stretches, in malls for instance, a wheel chair. Frankly, rather than risk losing the likelihood of drug approval, I have opted for the best-tested drug for which I qualify for financial help. Now, three other inteferons plus Avaonex are approved for Canada though not yet with Pharmacare [government assistance with drug costs] coverage. I might have been able to get private plan coverage for any of the others and still consider them options depending on how things go. For instance, I may require the pre-filled syringe available via Rebif if I can't see well enough to handle the Betaseron mix procedures, or if my right hand is too shaky. And a lot depends on the degree of symptom trouble I have. I'm not inclined to hop about from one drug to the other without a fair trial, which I think means six months.

My family is happy with the pro-drug decision, but we will see if it makes living with me even more problematic. Fevers, chills, flu symptoms, nausea, etc. could get hard, not to say messy. I'm not afraid of needles but it depends on the degree of pain. Every second day? Forever? Of course, a lot depends on the benefits. Let's hope so. Hope for the best for me!

Linda to Flora:

It seems to me MS is a very MSy ('messy') disease, unpre-dictable and so many possible/possibly new symptoms. I do hope your family will learn to cope as well as I know you will with your latest challenge. And maybe you'll be one of the lucky ones who don't suffer much at all with Betaseron; some report only a little discomfort at the injection site. Why, by the way, will you inject yourself, given how difficult it must be for you?

And now that you're on the drug program, I've forgotten just how difficult it was to get approved for it, i.e., for it to be covered by MSP (Medical Services Plan, our BC government coverage). Was that through the MS Clinic at UBC? What was the process?

And what supplements are you taking? Are you another in-house pharmacy, as I am? If you tell me yours, I'll tell you mine.

Flora to Linda:

Well, the first injection is over and side effects are minimal if not nil. After one day, what can one tell? So far, no flu-like symptoms or nausea, or headache. My regular, every day symptoms are a little bit worse. Harder to walk and more jittery. Or is the hot weather?

And later:

The injection procedures are hardly second nature yet. An interesting combination of memory problems (half a dose in one needle, push out the air for both needles, up-side down and smack it to get the bubbles out) and eye sight problems (what bubbles?) make the procedure the subject of much concentration. Next week I intend to travel. Get to an island in hot weather, shoot up in different surroundings, cope with worse symptom, if they get worse, and other interesting chal-lenges. Will keep you posted.

Linda to Flora:

My rule of thumb, developed with another MS buddy is "when in doubt, blame it on the weather." I take it one step further – "if you're in doubt about the culpability of the weather, blame it on menopause." Anything to take some of the mystery out of it all!

My neurologist has said for the last two years that "maybe next year we'll consider putting you on one of the drug programs," but I have been told that people like me who use a mobility aid for any distance walking, as I do, are not eligible. But I guess that was not the case or the research team has changed their idea of who might benefit.

Flora to Linda:

After about a week on Betaseron, I've discovered that other's definition of flu-like symptoms and even fever are entirely different from mine. At this point on half dose, I have worsening of MS symptoms and a very dry mouth in the morning. No nausea or headache. Not much of a site reaction at all. I take some Advil which I'm not convinced about, and more Tylenol, up to six a day. The theory is this will help the identifiable problems of increased shakiness in my right hand and increase in stiffness in the legs making it harder to walk even with the walker. Oddly, it's my left leg that is worse rather than the other which is usually less mobile. I have tried Baclofen again which isn't much use either (as yet) and in case of sleep problems have Atavan on hand for the first time in my life. But it doesn't seem to be the time to be a stoic.

Linda L. Ironside

I've done enough of that. Instead I meow a lot. But apart from more sleepiness, things aren't bad. I look forward to getting back to what was normal and then, who knows, maybe some improvement. Are we all skeptics? The medical people want to be very sure we don't have unrealistic expectations. I did ask the clinic nurse, if she had MS, would she take Betaseron? I didn't get an answer, which is fair I guess. She gave me lots of time to consider. And has been informative since, willing to repeat all info as required.

Three months later, Flora is still experimenting to find the best schedule for her injections, but can draw some conclusions.

Flora to Linda:

I have now completed three months on the treatment drug. I no longer have what is described as fever (wet upper lip and generally too warm when trying to sleep). I have learned to time injections more carefully – evenings but not too close to sleep time. The day after an evening injection is less good in terms of energy, but only slightly now. The most disappointing aspect is continued poor mobility. I understand this symptom will fade but as to when is very individual, and of course there are no promises. However, like the statisctically significant members of the study, I have had no relapses except what the drug itself has caused which I am sure is not officially a clinical relapse. Trust me to be having a harder time than usual with this. But there has been no decline into fatigue as I define it. Your comments about "less engagement" gave me pause. Would all this be easier if I rested more? I personally doubt it. In fact, I try for daily stretches as defined by my massage therapist. I suppose the best I can do is "do it my way." Got a notice today about more blood work. I presume that will be straightforward and unequivocal.

Linda to Flora:

I am looking forward to an extended period of time with no new challenges and not too much stimulation. (I sure sound old, don't I?) Good to hear you sounding so well, Flora, processing this phase of your life. Here we go into winter. After such a gorgeous autumn, we won't get much sympathy if we complain, will we?

> *Julie too is a "user", her drug of choice after some switching, Copaxone. She seems happy with it, and not too troubled by the common side effects like reactions where the injection is done and what people call flu-like symptoms.*

Julie to Linda:

I think in all the time we've been corresponding, I have confused you terribly in regard to my experiences with the ABC drugs. At different times, I have tried all three of the injectables, but at this time, and for the past twenty months, I have been on Copaxone. I am totally convinced that of the three, it is the only one that for me has made a difference. Let me back up and give you a chronological description of what I've experienced.

The first one that my neurologist, Dr. Desai, and I agreed to try was Betaseron. I did and adapted well to the subcutaneous injections every other day. I did experience some initial reaction with the typical flu-like feeling for the first several weeks. I had no real problem tolerating that because, to me it was a sign that my body's little army of T-Cells was on the offensive and was truly taking the newly introduced Interferon to war.

Of course, my positive attitude was busy at work making sure that I assumed that the drug would win. I'd have bet money on it, if I was a gambling soul. My MS exacerbations had been so regular and predictable spring and fall every year that I figured with Betaseron, the frequency would decrease. If it had done so, I would have been quite a happy camper, but it, in fact, did not. So, in the spring and fall of those two years, things were as they had been before Betaseron so my doctor and I made another decision. We felt that perhaps Avonex, in that it has a different atomic structure, would produce a more successful impact on my disease. The other positive aspect was felt by both of us to be the need to inject only once per week. Avonex is an intramuscular injection and could be more uncomfortable, but again my purely positive nature came surging forth. I thought: "Oh, Gee, if I travel, I have to pack so much less stuff!" So, I embarked on a period of weekly injections of Avonex. After 18 months, and three more exacerbations – fall, spring, fall, Dr. Desai and I had another of our discussions of the next move. In June of 1998, I began daily SubQ injections of Copaxone (Glatiramar Acetate). I have had no negative reactions to those injections, except for a little itching and redness at the injection site, but that has been relatively infrequent. Because of the fact that it's daily, I never forget, because it's something I do as part of my get up and get going routine.

The best part though for me is, I am absolutely positive that it has made a difference for me. In the fall of 1998, I had an exacerbation, but it was a weird one. I did not have any of the visual deterioration (that always led to gross imbalance and nausea) that I had in previous episodes. Now two things could be happening here. First, my disease process could be changing direction. Or, second, the Copaxone could actually be tempering the severity of my exacerbations and altering the frequency, so that I don't experience them in the same way as before. Whatever it is, I do not intend to mess with it. Copaxone and Julie Z are a team, and will continue to be for as long as I am convinced that it is helping, and for the last two years, MS for me has been less traumatic. I am also experiencing (since October of 19998) the monthly Solu-Medrol IV, which has stabilized me even more.

I do, by the way, have a little more deterioration in the use of my right hand. Grip strength and coordination for fine work like writing or holding small objects are diminished slightly. In May, after evaluation by my neurologist again, we may be considering the use of Plasmapheresis or Novantrone to tame the old immune system. Isn't it funny how in a world where everyone else is trying to build their immune systems up, we are trying to hold ours at bay, to keep them under control, so they'll stop attacking what they are not supposed to? What a pesky thing to have to deal with!

MS is so strange. With so many variables, and given the individuality of each of us, it is absolutely impossible to know what and if a particular intervention results in its desired outcome. Our positive attitudes usually serve us well, but sometimes, I think they also tend to baffle us. We like to expect the outcome we want, and so there we are thinking that's what we are experiencing, self-fulfilling prophecy or something like that, eh?

I need to collect my thoughts and organize them, and then I'll be contributing to the nasty bladder and bowel debate. What a "MeSsy" topic so to speak. Life would be so much easier if we didn't have to plan around those ugly episodes.

The saga continues. Flora decided to switch to Rebif for a couple of reasons less than a year later and reported on it after she'd made the adjustment.

Flora to Linda:

My switch to taking Rebif instead of Betaseron happened only about six weeks ago and I am working at recalling "why". The most important reason had to do with eyesight and problems seeing accurately the bubbles in the Betaseron syringe that needed to be cleared because they affected the quantity of the drug injected. This turned into a job for Alan, which he always did unless I was away or he was, in which case I did it myself and hoped for the best. I find the management of Rebif much easier and the actual injection is probably easier too. It's nice to have only three injections a week, leaving two days injection free. The schedule is therefore a little freer and more predictable, i.e. every Tuesday for instance. Because I chose not to use the autoinjector I have less to plan for and get the shot done in jig time whether at home or away.

And what is the effect? The good news is fewer negative results it seems. I still have trouble sleeping after a shot and poor walking ability generally. But today I was back trying the cane for part of the day. The walker is my mainstay most times and certainly in the evening. I am safer and it is certainly easier for Alan or others to sling into the car.

This is no change from the Betaseron days. On the other hand people remind me of how I am better than I was a while back. Not too definitive either way. Less fatigue than before is noticeable. But before Rebif? Anyway I do not feel worse than I was before either drug. So, by and large, I am happy with Rebif and feel optimistic about the treatment procedure. Remember the only real goal is fewer exacerbations per year and shorter ones if they happen. There are no promises and it is certainly not a cure. So I continue as was and feel grateful the drugs you mentioned are available virtually free most places in Canada and with my extended health in line, totally free for me in BC. If it slows the progression of the disease I am happy with it, shots and all. Keep your spirits up even though November is next.

A year after that, I had once again lost track of Flora and her drugs, so I prompted her for an update, and asked for the same from Julie, whose drug history has been more straightforward.

Flora to Linda:

I noticed discussion lately on the MS Canada newsgroup about treatment drugs and which to take or change to. As you know I started Betaseron August,1998. This was at the recommendation of my GP who had been following the research reports in medical journals. I checked some of the same information as had my adult children and got a lot of support for making the decision. I found the drug hard to get used to and relied heavily on the teaching assistance and then the telephone support of the MS clinic nurse at UBC.

Depression became a problem as did sleeping and I did a lot of shuffling of the time of injections. My trips out to UBC had started with my walker to get to various offices in the building complex. Next visits were with my wheel chair, which was simply easier and less tiring. My notes on symptoms indicate a particularly difficult first five or six months. This meant an increase in mobility problems and a distinct exacerbation at the end of January,1999. This included a short-lived increase in the band effect around my chest and general spasticity for one week or so. I think the Betaseron like the Rebif I am on now lives up to its reputation of keeping attacks down in number and shorter in duration.

I switched to Rebif after a year because the drug is available in pre-filled syringes, which eliminated the eyesight problems presented in the mixing procedure. It is easier to administer, which means I can do it all myself without working out Alan's schedule or planning other backup. I have not used the autoinject apparatus because I wanted to keep stuff and fuss down to a minimum and dealing with loading and carrying around the autoinject wasn't really required. There has been no site reaction to the Rebif injections, which I had after the start of the Betaseron. So in general they are not hard to do or hard to take. The special therapies nurse had told me about the possibility of having Rebif approved in Canada and covered by the provincial government in due course and when it was available I asked my neurologists to allow the switch.

Rebif is somewhat more expensive as a treatment drug though I am fully covered by my extended health plan through reimbursement after the first three or four months of the year.

It has proven to be a good drug decision for me. Remembering three days a week and always the same days isn't too hard rather than every second day with Betaseron. So it's Tuesday, Thursday or Saturday I plan an injection and the time of day is increasingly less critical. That said, I don't take them close to bedtime or I stay awake afterwards. So I usually take the syringe out of the fridge by five o'clock in the afternoon and do the injection by six. If this proves inconvenient any given day, I simply do it earlier while still at home. The last hour or two I have more trouble walking until after the shot. I am told this is a case of pre-injection jitters, which I find hard to credit because I have no concern about needles. I personally think this is too easy an explanation though I have learned that any physical response to emotions is possible in the MS world. But who knows and it isn't a major problem. And if I surprise myself and decide on an early afternoon injection, I have no early mobility problem. My four months on Rebif have not resulted in clearing up of the tingling, spasticity or loss of dexterity in my hands, which are benefits some people ascribe to Rebif but who knows what another five months may bring.

So, in summary, Rebif is definitely easier to administer and to tolerate and it may reduce the frequency and length of exacerbations which is the claim that research supports.

When it comes to drugs, people with MS are often private drugstores, using a variety of drugs to control various symptoms. Spasticity is one of the more serious effects of MS Julie and others have to cope with. New drugs to help deal with it are real cause for celebration – and a real disappointment when they don't work.

Linda L. Ironside

Julie to Linda:

Well, I've switched a couple of medications around in recent weeks, and so I'm experiencing new things. I mentioned starting Zanaflex before. I used to take Baclofen for spasticity, and the Zanaflex seems to be working much better. My urologist changed a bladder med (ProBanthene) that I was on to Ditropan XL, with which, after many months, I am very happy. I only take it once a day, not four times, as some do, and have no side effects.

Linda to Julie:

I guess that's the new Ditropan, industrial strength, is it? I took lots of Ditropan at one point, but no longer. I also drank Plantain tea, which was a help. Do you find you get so used to bladder troubles that you just fit that into your new sense of who you are, what you can do, what aids you need, etc. I've been wearing pads consistently for so long I'd feel naked without one, I think. I don't often need one, and maybe I could risk it without, but Kotex and I have built up a strong co-dependency. And I'm still incontinent for one day if I menstruate; that's an 'if' now rather than a 'when' as it is no longer a sure thing. Maybe you're lucky and are all finished with that? I think the hormones are terribly powerful; did I already tell you I'm using progesterone cream every day, which is as close to HRT (hormone replacement therapy) as I care to get.

Julie to Linda:

It was so-o-o nice talking to you on Sunday. Real voices add a lot to a conversation. I think I'm finally coming around to my normal state of existence . . . whatever that is. You know I told you I had a reaction to Zanaflex. I had a pretty noticeable drop in my blood pressure. My response was to simply change back to the medication I was previously on, Baclofen. With Zanaflex, you gradually increase to the effective dose, so that you don't have serious changes like that but, in spite of very slowly increasing my dose over several weeks, my blood pressure just wouldn't come out of the basement. I still wasn't at the dose that would work optimally on my spastic legs, so when I made the scheduled increase last week, I didn't expect to feel bad. I expected to feel GREAT! That wasn't the case, so as instructed, I made the switch back. I don't think my body wanted to do that, because I had three days of chills, nausea, and bad headache, followed by almost a week of feeling dull and drained (what's new?). This morning I seem to be wide-eyed and bushy tailed by comparison, so I think I've readjusted.

Over the past few days, the blood pressure has become stable once again, thank goodness. I didn't like feeling like I did. I know several people who are on Zanaflex who love it. I think I'm just one specimen who can't take it. I did well at the introductory doses, but WOW . . . that sure changed as we got going. I continue to use Copaxone daily and 1 gram of Solu-Medrol monthly by IV.

Last word on MS drugs from MS Word:

Did you know Spellchecker has a sense of 'humor', maybe even a sense of 'humour'? When it comes to drug treatments, Spellchecker suggests Avionics (Avonex) or Coppertone (Copaxone) and thinks all interferons are 'infernos.' Makes me want to produce typos just for the jokes they might produce! We shouldn't laugh until we've tried it, though. Has anyone injected Coppertone?

Talking about MS is not usually such a laugh.

EATIN' AND DRINKIN'

Diet. Nutrition. Food allergies. Words which become significant for anyone dealing with chronic illness. In the case of a disease where the cause is not yet known, some people hope to uncover dietary factors of the cause, while others want simply to ensure that their bodies are well enough nourished to achieve the optimum level of wellness. There have been many theories about MS and diet; it's a rich topic for discussion.

Flora to Linda:

Did you know about the food allergy clinic at VGH (Vancouver General Hospital)? Takes eight months to get in so I think I will call today.

Linda to Flora:

No, I didn't know about that. I wonder if the nurses at the MS Society do. I will check. My GP gave me a referral to an allergy specialist, who was recommended by someone else with MS; he's also covered by MSP, so I'm very happy. I'll see him in early June as I'll be away when he has room in May. I was so pleased I got the referral, not only because it makes it all easier, but also because it shows my GP and I are working as a team.

Several years ago I changed my diet considerably, opting for an amalgam of changes which had been recommended – no gluten, low fat, no dairy. It was surprisingly easy to adjust to my new regimen, since I love rice. But I am human; I do occasionally have food memories (AKA cravings).

Linda to Flora:

Well, I think the change in diet has really taken hold. More than I want it too sometimes. Like today.

I was craving something gooey, sweet, delicious, a dough-nut or a cream puff or one of the wheat-based goodies I haven't indulged in for so long, the kind of comfort food I would resort to when I was feeling out of sorts. So I planned to get one of these delights in the health food store where I was going to pick up some balsamic vinegar and homeopathic sinus pellets, a trip I make every few months. After picking up the things on my list, I went to the bakery section to satisfy that craving. But when the clerk asked me what I wanted, I heard myself ask, "Have you got anything that's gluten-free?" I came away with a muffin made with rice flower. No cream, no fatty sauce, no icing. And one part of my brain, the freedom-loving, rebellious side was sad that the disciplined, reasonable, obedient brain had the upper hand yet again. I suppose the memories of how I felt after the last "gluten orgy" were too fresh for that brain to ignore.

And the taste? Dry, as rice flour is, I find. Mealy, like a mouthful of corn meal. A raisin here or there to alleviate the sameness and give a hint of a pastry shop goodie. But this was your basic prison muffin, a serious food item. I washed it down with a can of Pepsi, just on the edge of verboten land, and definitely gluten-free.

Flora to Linda:

I would really like to know what happened when you gave in to gluten gluttony. I seem to be able to have even wheat, only a little to be cautious without any effect. What would I expect – headache, gut ache, guilt for deserting the side? And was that diet Pepsi?

Now sugar I do feel. An unhappy tummy.

You see, I am a literal soul. You have a fun episode and I come up with how come, how much and what happened. And by the way, what is a homeopathic pellet? I would want to know what you use for sinus treatment. Does it work and can you buy it without RCMP (Royal Canadian Mounted Police) permission? I can see indices growing.

Linda to Flora:

It is so much more difficult to be specific, give details, but necessary, I know. I think I'm a person who likes to live in the forest rather than in the trees, if you know what I mean. Always prone to making vague generalizations.

Anyway, back to the subject at hand. My first adverse reaction to gluten after I'd been gluten-free for some time was after I treated myself and had pizza – and not just one slice. I felt so tired afterward! I remember thinking, "This is good! A negative reaction like this will serve to remind me of why I'm doing this, and keep me on track." A month or so ago, after I just threw all caution to the wind and indulged in fats *and* gluten, I could feel my whole system slow down, basically grind to a halt – lethargy and fatigue I usually associate with an exacerbation. Again, a not-so-friendly reminder.

As for the Pepsi, no it was not diet. I drink about three cans op pop a year, so seldom subject my body to that junk. But I am not counting calories or watching my intake of sugar per se. I'm not big on sweets now, though, so don't take in a lot. I miss fresh bread more than I miss cookies. But every once in a while, like the muffin day I told you about, I really crave sweet, such as ice cream or a chocolate bar or a gooey doughnut. Maybe I'm pregnant?

As for homeopathic pellets – that's my term for them. They're small, round, and I take several at once. I've noticed lately that the regular drug stores (Shopper's Drug Mart, London Drugs) are carrying certain homeopathic remedies for common ailments like sinus, cold, fatigue, etc. Homeocan is the brand name of the ones I buy there. I find them very effective for a long-standing sinus problem, which is one of the few complaints I have which I can't link to MS. I'm also sending them to my mother whose genes are the origin of my sinus troubles. She also reports positive results, and she has it much worse than I do.

How about you, Flora? Would you recommend a gluten-free diet? Any other changes in diet? What about the allergist you were going to?

Meanwhile, I'll stick to my rice in a bowl, not in my bread.

Flora to Linda:

I haven't kept to any gluten-free diet mostly because the weight loss I experienced made it seem a poor idea. I had taken some weight off in early 1996 but once my exacerbation started that November, I lost forty pounds. I've stabilized now but it was worrisome. But I became very sensitive to foods and spices. Over time I have learned to avoid balsamic vinegar, which causes a coughing and sneezing fit and makes breathing difficult; chocolate in large amounts and strawberries give the same reaction. All this is new and quite startling.

The only reaction I got to an allergy test was tofu, which I have learned to keep minimal. Alan developed a great recipe for miso soup which we both liked and ate three or four days in a row. First day was fine, then after lunch I become terribly weak and could barely make it to bed. Half an hour later all was relatively fine. The chocolate/strawberry combination put me in bed for half a day. And I ate only four – honest!

I stay away from pickled foods and meats, never have liked raw fish, or perhaps the idea of it, and while I enjoy shrimp, they must be fresh and very well washed. These reactions might have to do with preservatives. The main lesson clearly is to pay attention to your reactions to food, don't overdo anything in case you find yourself in trouble and tread cautiously. I am now definitely sensitive to foods I happily chomped through in earlier years but I am not as reactive as some of my cousins or my mother. I have returned beef to my diet after shunning it for years. My preference is free range, which means no antibiotics. The same applies to chicken. We eat a lot of fish and put a heavy emphasis on fruits and green vegetables. Do I sound like the Canada Health Rules? I do not, however, drink milk but use Rice Dream instead with my cereal. I use butter and cheese but prefer hard cheese and not the creamy.

This response seems to involve unending detail but my diet is really quite straightforward and easy to manage.

A Mystery Show like MS naturally leads to lots of different theories about treatment as well as cause. And the stories of people who have recovered to some extent are both encouraging and confusing, as there is so little which can be easily generalized. In my search for what will help me, what my body needs, I have tried a variety of alternative therapies. But none quite so never-thought-you'd-catch-me-doing-this as the following.

Linda to Flora:

Spent a couple hours this afternoon with someone trying to convince me I should drink a glass of my own urine each day. Sent me away with yet another book on it, and more tales of the wondrous effects. Now and then backed up by her partner, a sculptor who worked in the studio while Nori and I talked. She too is an artist, she too has MS. Sometimes I resent the framework of my life so often spelling out MS. But I don't when it puts me in touch with people like her. And when I get to read e-mail from Kenya, as I do on an MS newsgroup. C'est la vie.

Yes, I did try it, for a while (I can hardly believe it myself). Who am I to reject what was good for Gandhi? It may have helped me, but in the end was just too impractical to become a habit. The books, by the way, provided very compelling, researched arguments and testimonials.

CHECKING OUT
COMPLEMENTARY MEDICINES

Over 50,00 Canadians and 350,000 Americans have this disease, with no known cause and no cure and not even a universal, dependable treatment. It is not surprising that many of us have turned to alternative/complementary medicines for relief of our symptoms. TCM (Traditional Chinese Medicine) is my alternative medicine of choice, but there's also massage therapy, plus Reiki, Yoga, and other physical stimulation techniques, mercury amalgam removal, bee stings , in fact, a host of other means seeking to develop our wellness. None of them can be discounted, no matter how zany they sound, because they wouldn't be talked about if they hadn't helped someone, somewhere. Flora, Julie, and I have all had a dip in this pool, without renouncing what conventional medicine offers. This has led to some very interesting experiences.

Linda to Flora:

Results I experienced when I started TCM (acupuncture, moxibustion, foot reflexology) five years ago were dramatic. I kept a graph at that time to record my general feeling of wellness. At the end of a year, my lowest point was where my highest was to start. All very subjective, of course. The treatments once a week are now helping keep me stable, keeping further inflammation at bay, and dealing with any incidental symptoms that pop up from time to time, like pain or discomfort here or there, a bad week for balance, bladder on strike, etc. And now I also do the moxibustion at home every day or two. My energy is better than it was, my thinking is clearer, my short-term memory better. I still do, however, use a cane for my short walks in the park and a scooter to get me there, unlike other patients who have been able to put their wheelchair in storage.

It doesn't work for everyone. A key to my success with it has been my unfaltering faith in Chinese medicine ever since I was diagnosed in hospital in Beijing. If you don't believe it will work, your mind will sabotage the best efforts of any medical practitioner, western or Chinese. Another key has been the regularity of treatments, and the length of time. TCM offers no quick fix. To start, I had treatments three times a week. Expensive? Yes. But I long ago accepted the fact that I was one of those unfortunate people who dare not take their health for granted, for whom health care costs are part of the monthly budget, like food. It's an investment I have found paid off – I really hated a life without joy, dragging my you-know-what through the motions of living. Another key is finding a well-trained practitioner. Many have no real medical training; many have no real understanding of MS.

I sound like a true believer, don't I? But even after years of treatments, I still am very aware I am allowing, even encouraging, someone to treat my body like a pincushion. And there are limits to what I can mentally accept.

Linda L. Ironside

Linda to Julie:

I just came back from acupuncture and am still nervous. In the past, I've had needles put in my head, my belly, my feet, my hands, and of course, my legs and arms. I am very used to it all and there's more comfort involved than discomfort. But I have to say I got a start today when I happened to mention just "by the way" that the ophthalmologist examined the optic nerve in my left (most affected side) eye and found there's been optic atrophy. Since I have not noticed a deterioration in vision, I wasn't particularly alarmed. But when I told Dr. Ma, she immediately countered with, "We've had a lot of success improving vision." My mind immediately went racing off to threats of 'needles in your eye.' I watch too many gangster movies, I guess. But she is very good at what she does, and understands how to deal with the common trepidation patients feel. Before I could work up a sweat, I had one additional needle in my cheek, and one in my eyebrow. Both pinched a bit going in, but once in, were fine. Will it help? Don't know, but I'm willing to give it a try. She says the stimulation to that channel will help prevent further atrophy, and may reduce the inflammation of the nerve. I think if I can buy into the TCM as valid, then it wouldn't make sense to say, "Okay, but only for the bladder, legs, etc., not for the eyes."

My reaction to her suggestion that needles would help was, come to think of it, similar to that of others when I tell them I place burning herbs on my head (the moxibustion). It's all relative, isn't it? I'll be asking her to continue the extra needles as long as she thinks it may help.

By chance, Julie also had had experience with acupuncture, but she kept it in the family.

Julie to Linda:

My experience with acupuncture was one three week-long episode of two treatments per day. My brother-in-law, Mike's younger brother, is a practitioner of Chinese Medicine. His office is in Tampa, Florida. Michael and I were visiting his mother in Hudson, a little bit north of Tampa, so it was an excellent opportunity to visit with both her and "little brother". He spent some time with me collecting history and symptom information, and we decided that the experience of acupuncture would benefit me in a number of ways. The goals that we were working toward were several. The most significant of them was to bring about a general improvement in the feeling of well-being. My energy level was very poor at the time (I was still trying to maintain my full time responsibilities at the hospital). My body was riddled with minor aches and pains, I think now, mostly due to sheer exhaustion from trying to keep up with life as usual, the old this-ain't-gonna'-get-me-down denial phase of coming to grips with MS. It was two and a half years after diagnosis. I was also experiencing severe pain in my lower back when I'd wake up in the morning. I now attribute this to spasticity, and definitely related to MS. This is pain that I would periodically experience, and can recall as far back as when I was in my twenty's. This is why I am so convinced that I had actually been an MSer for many years before I was motivated to seek diagnosis. My appetite was not up to par, and I was losing weight as a result. Bill (Dr. Zuby) had his work cut out for

him, and I was fully prepared to accept any and all sugges-
tions and treatment methods he was to recommend. We
agreed to two trips into Tampa per day for acupuncture, some
herbal therapy, and daily massage therapy.

Well, in terms of immediate response, I felt wonderful.
The objectives were met. The general aches and pains and
overall fatigue were overcome within a few days. The back
pain, that I found to be very difficult to cope with, was reduced
gradually until by the time we returned to Michigan, I was no
longer experiencing it. I'll come back to the back pain later,
because there's more to the ongoing treatment of that. My
appetite responded to something. I've never been completely
sure of what. What I mean is: I'm sure that the herbal mix that
he had prescribed for me was a factor. The appetite, though,
had declined as I had begun to feel lousy. The feeling lousy was
what led me to treatment with him in the first place. As I
generally began to feel better during my stay in Florida, my
appetite returned to a more normal state. I don't know that I
can attribute that return to any one form of treatment. I think
more so to the combination of all factors and methods. Bill
also taught me some Yoga "Asanas", and we practiced those
until I was able to return home equipped to continue them
here, and I do. The stretching and improved tone that resulted
have been invaluable in many ways, but the biggest effect was
the reduction and almost complete absence of my nasty back
pain. I often feel now that the Yoga and resulting maintenance
of muscle tone and balance are at the root of my back pain
reduction.

Of course, Bill recommended that I follow through with
acupuncture and massage therapy. He also hoped that I would
continue with the herbal treatment, and would dispense them
to me from his office in Florida if I continued to do so. I'm sure
he's more than a little disappointed in me for not following

through, but as I've said to you before, I am a rather traditional medicine connoisseur. I am managing my MS with a number of pharmaceutical agents, and I have a serious concern about the potential negative effect of adding non-trialed (clinical trials) agents, the herbal treatments, to the medicines I take. I'm afraid that one will negate the effect of the other, or worse yet, they might have a synergistic effect and produce some reaction for which I'm not prepared.

Anyway, the whole experience was a good one. I loved the outcome of the acupuncture, and would probably continue it here if I could: a) afford it as my insurance doesn't cover it, and b) know for sure that it was doing something positive on an ongoing basis. In general, I feel as though my MS is being very well managed via the traditional methods that I utilize, and so I just plan to continue on that path, with Yoga now being a part of my life, not in a major way, but truly benefiting me in terms of almost non-existent back pain. That is a marvelous outcome, for which I am very grateful to my brother-in-law!

Moxibustion is another TCM treatment which is fairly simple and rather fun to talk about. It involves burning some dried herb (mugwort) on your head, or any other acupuncture point, for that matter, cut from a roll, which looks like a small cigarette, and set ever so gently on a bed of ginger, which has been placed on the desired spot. The fun comes when people come by and see me sitting in front of a mirror burning something on my head and maybe fanning it – a Woodstock dropout?

Linda to Flora:

I'm going to resist the temptation to open a note to you with a comment about the weather. Nope, I won't do it. We both know it's dreadful, so it would be masochistic to go over it all again, right?

So, back to my favorite topic with you, MS remedies. You mentioned that you tried moxibustion at one point, didn't you? Did you do it yourself at home? I forget, of course.

I tried it for the first time this morning, but I definitely have to check out my technique. My acupuncturist suggested I do it to provide more stimulation to the head than I can get at my weekly treatments with her. I had mentioned my balance is getting worse. She asked a few questions to ensure something else wasn't involved, and then said to try the moxi she had given me some time ago and I had stored away. The balance thing really scares me, and I will do anything I can to slow its decline. But no fresh ginger in the place, and I had to use old stuff. But the moxi smoked down to ash as it was meant to. It felt very much the same as when she puts a needle in that spot. Of course, I had someone help and stay around for the ten to fifteen minutes it took to do its work.

Did you? Do you? Why? Why not?

Flora to Linda:

Yes, I did moxibustion at the acupuncturist for about a year and then at home for maybe six months. It was a help when done weekly in terms of energy particularly. I stopped when I found I got such a buzz from the process it kept me too wound up. I haven't tried it in conjunction with Betaseron – that also keeps me fairly hyper particularly on injection days. Fresh ginger is essential as I remember, and having it burn to ash in about twenty minutes is normal, if you want to keep it on for that long. I used the non-smell type most recently that can be held close like a cigar. The ash is tapped off also like a cigar. It's one of the aspects of treatment I miss and will get back to weekly as soon as I can.

Have you tried the non-smelling moxi? Otherwise your home smells distinctly smelly like it could be you are burning an illegal substance!

I certainly haven't been impressed with every alternative treatment I tried.

Linda to Julie:

What do you know about so-called "psychic healers"? I had seen people referred to that way but had never really read much on anyone. So I was fascinated when Nori, who had seen a short blurb on a psychic healer in this area, urged me to go with her to see what he could do. I try to keep my mind open to all forms of treatment, at least until I have personal experience or a good reason not to look further. So off we went!

While he worked on Nori, my friend, I sat and read the letters and testimonials satisfied clients had written tales of the wonderful benefit they had felt. These were all nicely collected in big albums sitting on the coffee table in the waiting room, which I thought was very clever, even helpful. But his preparation for the actual hands-on was a little too clever for my tastes, covering all the bases. "Don't know when it will happen", "Might take a few sessions", "Can't predict" etc., points which I didn't think needed to be stated. He did more telling than asking, which is not my idea of how a healer who tries to heal a person rather than a sickness works. The treatment itself consisted of the patient lying on a bed, fully clothed, covered by a blanket, in a semi-private alcove while a tape of Pachebel's Canon played. He held his hands just above certain parts of the body, repeating that he didn't have a plan to this, and couldn't say where he would hold his hands, except that he would not put them near any private areas. After a half-hour or so of this, he left the client to lie alone, eyes closed, with music playing, for another thirty minutes.

Then he reappeared, and asked what I felt, what sensations went through my body, etc. These were usually "quite common" or "very interesting". I told him I felt a wave of heat flowing over me. He asked the direction, and I told him, from right to left. He was very interested in that and I felt like an A student for a moment, until I mentioned that the small, portable heater on the floor was to the right of the bed. When he had finished with the healing hands and left me to lie quietly, he went out and engaged in conversation with Nori, which was perfectly audible to me, and sort of broke the spell of Pachebel. When I later told him that it was very distracting to hear them talking, he explained that it really didn't matter, as by that time, any benefit I was going to receive I already had.

This guy was a used car salesman of the first order. I also believe that he is able to help people. He builds confidence in his healing power with his talk, then promotes total relaxation for an extended period. Very powerful healing tools.

I think we're all interested in finding what will help us, and I recognize it is very individualistic. I've been impressed by the people who seem to recover a lot of health and mobility after years of using a wheelchair, etc. Two of the things often mentioned are massage and meditation. I'm doing both of these now, but it's too early to tell if there's any stable, continuing benefit. And I'm still continuing the acupuncture, of course. But, boy oh boy, do you ever have to cling to a strong belief! I figure it's pretty impossible for me to know exactly what is doing what for me. As long as I have a strong belief that something is beneficial, is helping me be at my optimum functioning level, I will continue. I'd like to find some way of improving my balance, which is the one symptom that has shown the most decline, even while others, such as bladder, energy, fatigue have improved. I think strengthening my thigh muscles would help, and am trying to exercise them a little each night. I found that I overdid it the first night and had jelly thighs the next day.

Julie to Linda:

I've never tried a psychic healer, not my style at all, but you are so right when you say, "We're all interested in finding what will help us, and recognize it is very individualistic." Another statement of yours: " Boy oh boy, do you ever have to cling to a strong belief! I figure it's pretty impossible for me to know exactly what is doing what for me. As long as I have a strong belief that something is beneficial, is helping me be at my optimum functioning level is so-o-o-o very true of all of us. I think my diligent pursuit of the medical intervention thing is strongly rooted in my own experience of working in the medical field, and the trust I've developed over the years in that arena.

There are also a score of ideas (conflicting, of course) about exercise and muscle stimulators for MS. Passive exercisers, machines that move your legs or arms for you, seem ideal. Simply strap yourself in, turn the machine on, and away you go, with next to no effort required of your muscles. But it's not the ideal solution because, as we forget at our peril, our problem starts with the nerves, not the muscles, and passive exercises can r-e-a-l-l-y tire the nerves. As I found out.

Linda to Flora:

This disease never lets us relax, does it? There's always so much I want to discuss with you about MS. It's so good to have someone who understands what I'm talking about and gives me feedback! What is the current state of your treatment regimen? Do you do any meditation? Ever have? What alternative medicine are you still using? Send me all your secrets, please, Flora.

Flora to Linda:

I like the idea of meditation but can't claim seriously to have tried it. Massage is a fine practice and I have been to various physiotherapists. I intend to start acupuncture again this fall and found in the past that it definitely helped my balance and mobility. Or I could remind myself that was several years ago, maybe before my MS had progressed as much. Healing touch is a real phenomenon, and I have just begun the Feldenkrais

Method, with its emphasis on "functional integration" and "awareness through movement." It seems like a very gentle form of bodywork but claims to have more to do with reprogramming the brain. So after all of one treatment by a person who is also a physiotherapist I was impressed with the effect and will attend for treatment for a while and go to classes weekly for eight weeks (at minimal cost) via the Vancouver School Board. Keep tuned, seems like a nice combination of mind based bodywork and body focused movement. Very gentle, very soothing. But psychic healing it isn't, which sounds too much like somebody else trying for control.

Linda to Flora:

I would love to know more. Do you have the patience to answer a couple questions? What happens during a session? Is it done in a class or one-on-one? What benefit do you feel you get from it? How expensive is it?

And functional integration sounds very interesting. I've never heard you mention that. Does it go by any other name? What do you do? How did you find the practitioner you go to? How long have you been doing it?

I'm sure that this is one of those holistic therapies, which seems the only treatment type to make sense. You must be pretty busy with appointments. A response will be most welcome whenever you find the time. The only treatment I've used lately which I can highly recommend is a sunny day, like today. Can't beat it!!

Glad you're still questing.

Flora to Linda:

Yes, I really like my Feldenkrais Method work. Functional Integration, in my case, is sessions held in a physiotherapist's office. These are one hour, plus an extra quarter hour in the beginning. Cost is sixty dollars each session. The therapist was suggested via a counseling contact I had last fall. There are therapists who use this method who can be located via the Feldenkrais Guild of North America. Local practitioners can also be found via school board classes or at community centres. The cost of my classes totaled fifty-seven dollars for eight classes. They last for one and one half hours and include maybe fourteen or sixteen people.

There are many books in the library by Moshe Feldenkrais and others who write about his method. His best-known work is "Awareness Through Movement," and the title defines the process. The classes and the sessions help you learn to move with minimum effort and to shift from habitual patterns of movement to new mind-body connections. For me it has improved balance and led to very deep relaxation as well as positive changes in breathing. There is an emphasis on self-scanning and therefore being aware of the differences each day in your condition. I have been amazed to find I can relax completely with no tremors or pain. I don't know how the method works except that it is not muscle-based, repetitive or hard on the body. It seems to tie to changes in the brain and gentle ways of triggering those changes. I find it hard to explain but experience it as pleasant, supportive and stress reducing. Does this make any sense?

People with MS can no longer, as many still can, take their health for granted. It takes our discipline, our concentration and, our money. Treatments, conventional or supplemental, are often costly, even after the health plans contribute. Some of them are out of the question for many people, which is very unfortunate, because every new treatment, conventional or alternative, brings hope. That is reason enough to keep looking, and trying.

GETTING AROUND

MS is, in the public perception ('mis'conception), auto-matically associated with a wheelchair. And while mobility is a major problem that most people with MS have to deal with, some people don't have this particular feature of the disease at all, and for others, it may not be the most troubling. Personally, I find the problems at the other end of my body – i.e. muddle-headedness, forget-fulness, and son on, much more frustrating. However, Flora, Julie and I all do struggle with walking and have the full complement of aids – canes, walkers, scooters, crutches and wheel chairs. Legs are definitely more convenient. When you get into the car, for example, there they are, right under you, no need to collapse them, pack them up and throw them into the back. But using a mobility aid is certainly better than the alternative, being immobile. When you're stuck in the house, dependent on others to get out, a scooter or motorized chair is a solution, not a problem. As with anything in life, there is a whole range of experiences, delights and frustrations with getting around.

For Flora, of course, part of the problem is her extremely limited vision, but that doesn't seem to hold her back much. In fact, as she thinks about the new home she and hubby will move into, she tells me not about what she'll have inside but rather, how she will get out.

Flora to Linda:

You gave me pause with your comment on restricted lifestyle. Of course that's the way to describe how things are at the moment. Limitations of disability and fatigue impact every aspect of life. But I find I am constantly looking for substitutes. I have found, for instance, that asking someone to drive me someplace gets me where I want to go. But so does Handidart, admittedly with a good bit of planning. Haven't used it much of late and I miss it. It has a yes-you-can feel and so have the people I meet on the busses. The difficulties of going two or three municipalities away and back are daunting sometimes but that is a major bonus to the move we have on the horizon.

I shall get back to my old shopping district – post office, ATM, health store, shopping for presents, lunch out, library, and more. I will depend on personal power but the district I have in mind has no hills or at least it once had no hills when the world was flatter and more accessible. My major limitation will be intersections. "Is that light red?" But it is busy enough that there will always be other people to take a cue from. Having auditory signals are in fact rare. Which raises the question of whether or not I get a scooter. Then going up or down even slight rises would be easier. In a wheelchair it can be tough or downright scary. I admire your transportation skills and ability to get about with a scooter in tow.

Linda to Flora:

Now this I can relate to, the never-ending quest for balance with life in general and with MS in particular. I still wonder if

I started using a scooter too soon. But when I think what it allowed me to do, i.e., keep working, the answer is pretty clear. I could still walk ten years ago, better than I do now, but those long corridors at the college sapped strength/energy I wanted to use in the classroom. Our decisions regarding the use of aids are not unlike any decision we make in life, I guess. We weigh the pros and the cons and one side wins. The only difference is the added difficulty of remaining rational when the issue is, or seems at the time, so vital. I'm turning more and more over to my sub-conscious. "Here are the facts as I know them; sort through them, decide what's best and let me know. I'll be the one in bed."

Flora to Linda:

I have been to two large gatherings lately and was using my chair at both. I have learned that people may not know if I am just behind them, either because they glanced over their shoulder and of course didn't see me or because I am too quiet (no clicking heels?) And suddenly I very nearly have a lapful of company. I am used to standing tall – 5 foot 10.5 inches – and being someone who was hard to miss. I use "excuse me" frequently, which at a noisy party has no effect. Should I tug on clothing like little kids have learned to do? Should I use a bell? Whistle? Or I can give a smart nudge with the chair, which isn't so friendly. Probably all equally startling.

At the other event, a smart director sited a large, heavy bench for me to sit near so people could talk to me at eye level. I appreciated this and I'm sure they were glad to sit down for a while.

Personal space is now different. If someone knows I am low vision, I can have a face shoved in my face without warning. There are some savvy folks who don't try to wave from across the room, but approach, introduce themselves if necessary and stay nearby for a conversation. The ones who get it right are so appreciated!

The advantage is that I can move around a room, if not too crowded. Do you have any similar experiences while on your scooter?

Linda to Flora:

Interesting comments, Flora. If I think about scootering, I realize that the funny thing is that I feel less disabled than when I'm walking with a cane. Yet, to most people who see me, it's the opposite. A person in a scooter is treated quite differently. I have trouble with the fact that eye contact is not easy with me down so much lower than them. If I'm with a walker or two, I might just be ignored. Grrr! On my scooter I have more energy to be sociable, to chat, but am being cut out of the loop. On the other hand, when I'm walking, I have no desire to chat, exchange niceties, pass the time of day. I want only to get where I'm going and SIT DOWN. People are generally nervous around me in the scooter (it moves!) or are unnecessarily solicitous, leaving me a much wider berth than required. But I enjoy scootering, testing my driving skills down crowded aisles, passing people with a little beep on the street. I'm having so much fun, nothing much detracts from it. Maybe because for so long I didn't use one and any outing was characterized first and foremost by difficulty. Fun? What was fun about that? I've had a scooter at home here for three years now, but the novelty still has not worn off. Of course, I still drive as well, but that is work (the walking involved when I get there, not the driving itself).

Your comments made me realize just how much there is for people to adapt to, I mean those who are not in the wheel-chair. But isn't it good to be at this point in the evolution of disability, to be part of the public awareness process. Who is going to be talking about this in twenty years? Who was talking about it twenty years ago? Our timing is good, Flora!

And if we drive, we have those nice handicapped placards to hang on the rear view mirror so we can avail ourselves of the special parking spots set aside for handicapped drivers. That is, if an able-bodied driver hasn't taken it. Do you know about the stickers you can buy from Abilities Foundation in Toronto, the people who produce the magazine, which you can stick to someone's windshield? "No, I am not disabled! I just took this spot to show that I don't give a damn and am very, very important." White lettering on an orange background. I am very careful where I use them, as I wouldn't want to 'sticker' someone who was not totally deserving.

Another trick I like is boxing the offending car in, parking behind them when their side is also blocked. If I'm in luck, they return to the car before I get into the shop and I can call out to them, "I'll just be a minute!" And it seems there's always something in the shop to catch my attention, causing me to dally just a minute longer. I once had a woman come in after me and beg me to come and move my car. Now that's what I call a teachable moment! I haven't had much success, though, with talking to people. I don't know what to say to an able-bodied driver who can watch a single, disabled woman come over, then offer no apology, only the timeworn excuses. When someone is genuinely sorry and apologizes, on the other hand, I am so touched I want to take them home.

Flora to Linda:

This is a big public education task. Some people think because of the graphic on the parking tag it apples only to people actually using wheel chairs at the time. Or it apples only if the driver is the one who is disabled. Access to parking spaces, particularly prime ones, is an emotional issue for lots of able-bodied folks if much less justifiably. Our parking tag is mine but used on our car, which I do not now drive. If people don't notice me getting out of the car (or staying in it) they can assume my husband (walking smartly off to get groceries) is a "mis-user" of the parking tag privilege. Takes some interpretation on occasion.

Linda to Flora:

The worst case I have seen was a handicapped stall in a restaurant parking lot, on an incline that was difficult for me to walk up. You drove in off a very busy road (Kingsway in Vancouver) and up a steep incline to the handicapped stall, right in front of the door (very nice). But anyone trying to extricate themselves from a vehicle and into a wheel chair would be at risk of rolling backwards down the slope into the traffic (not so nice). Another case of provisions being made for people who have a disability, but an attendant or companion is required. Like the washrooms which require someone else to handle the doors so I can get in to use the specially marked toilet stall. Making life easier for helpers, but not yet making it possible for people with a disability to be independent. The playing field may be not as slanted as it was, but it's not yet level.

Linda L. Ironside

As is so often the case, people with a disability are often our own worst enemy. We can hardly help others learn an enlightened attitude if we ourselves are still living in the old stereotypes and fail to behave as independent, whole people.

Linda to Julie:

Now for an old type of interaction failure, one I thought we'd gotten beyond: I'm at the airport with my sister, Susan. I am in a wheelchair, as the distances are extensive. One of the airline ticket agents is checking on my plans and asks Susan something about me, as if I were not there or could not speak for myself. "How many bags does she have?"

Now, the shocking part is that I didn't even catch it at the time; Susan later told me what she had said. Is that because I was tired and not focused? Because I was happy to leave all the details to Susan and tune out? Or maybe because there's a wheelchair mentality which I too readily adopt quite unconsciously. I turn my life over to those around me all too willingly, and am happy to play passive possum for a spell. Am I a collaborator in this denial of my presence, my identity? On my scooter I am very assertive, erring more on the side of too much than not enough. Truth is, I feel very different in a wheelchair being pushed around by someone. If I could wheel myself, I think I'd feel different.

While we're on the subject, why are wheelchairs always black? Scooters are coloured. I see in the photos you sent that yours is blue; mine is maroon. Who ever said that the image of wheelchairs should never change from the serious, dark, tragic picture they used to present? Why does no one come out with a wheelchair with a variety of coloured backs, which a person could switch to be colour-coordinated with clothing or mood? Why, Julie, why?

Julie to Linda:

I didn't know the black wheelchair rule: I have one that is bright yellow . . . was trying not to be sad that I had to use it, but instead, to feel happy that I had one to use! Anyway, since Mike developed a cold on Thursday, and his mother, at the lake, should not be exposed to anything like that if it can be avoided, we stayed home. She'll be leaving for Florida on Wednesday with a neighbor of hers who also goes to Florida for the winter.

I seem to be having so much trouble following through with promises. I really shouldn't make promises. They are born of good intentions, but stuff keeps happening or as is the case in the past couple weeks, my routine has not been very routine. Nothing bad going on, just got busy, and when that happens, I nap in down time instead of going to the computer. I've been engaged a little bit in activities with the kids, the zoo, a couple of picnics, and just some real serious bonding time. Three of the five of them have birthdays right around now, Cole yesterday and the twins on July 7th. We are all having one of our backyard barbeque get-togethers on Sunday, so we're making a birthday party out of it, balloons and all with three cakes and fun.

I'm working on arranging a seminar for another consultant . . . doing some serious marketing for him. Been identifying target names, and arranging his brochure. So, anyway, I'm learning new stuff again. I'm wearing the hat of "Julie the

conference planner and marketing rep.".". It's a new hat. I hope
I do it right.

Julie's response to my previous comments;

You said, "I just may have to come to Hawaii or Greece or
Mexico. My, my, wherever shall I go?" Wouldn't that decision
be a fun one to make, I'll be your luggage, better get my pass-
port up to current, I don't want to slow you down when you get
rolling.

About the walker. I've traveled with it several times and
never had any damage (luck?). I put a luggage tag on it so that
if it becomes separated from the place it's supposed to be,
maybe it could find me again. I did, when I traveled to Cali-
fornia a couple years ago, board the plane with it. I didn't have
anyone with me to carry purse and coat, etc., and I took it with
me to walk through the airport. Actually, that was far too much
walking, with or without the walker. On the return trip, I asked
for wheelchair assistance. The man pushed my chair while I
pushed the walker with my luggage on it. Quite a picture, eh?

I went out to dinner last night with some friends that I
used to work with and I'm going out tonight with a longtime
friend who I don't get to see very often. I think we call these
social whirls. It sure used to take a whole lot heavier schedule
than that to get me thinking I was busy.

Hope you're doing well and feeling well. Next week on
Wednesday, Mike and I are leaving for a few days in Wiscon-
sin, poking around the area where my early relatives settled in
the 1850s. Then we'll drive through the Upper Peninsula of
Michigan for a few days and take care of my mother-in-law for
a few more.

Scooters are fun, like big toys. Canes are a very different matter. And most people don't realize that I need help when I'm using a cane, more than I do when I'm on my scooter. But sometimes people can see my need and just intuitively know what to do. They are the ones who turn a challenge into a rewarding, enjoyable outing.

Linda to Julie:

It was nice to hear from you on the topic of helpful strangers, as I recently also had a lovely experience with people I'd never seen before. You also wrote about the difficulty getting through a door someone is holding for you. MS just doesn't like doors, I guess, as I also have trouble occasionally, when someone is 'helping' me. I use the door for balance, one hand on the door handle, one on the cane. Some kind soul comes along, opens it wide and holds it for me; I won't let go of the handle so am sort of dragged along. I'm not articulate at the best of times when I'm standing, but in this caper, I am reduced to a very awkward, pitiful cry of anguish. The Samaritan, of course, has no idea what is wrong; most people do not realize the importance of door handles in keeping a person standing. Another troublesome door is the locked one from our underground parking. I walk up to it, lunge at it actually on a bad day and grab hold of the handle for balance while I do the key thing. Woe betide us both if some innocent is heading to the garage and opens the door from the other side while I am clinging to it like a life raft. I'm sure I'm a real sight to behold, gamely trying to cling to the door as they gamely try to open it. Do my eyes betray my feeling of terror? How did I get onto the subject of doors?

Linda L. Ironside

Let me talk about people I haven't terrorized. A couple weeks ago, I went down to Steveston, just south of Vancouver, to take a little boat tour of Cannery Channel, the area on the Fraser River where there used to be many fish canneries, and where there still are lots of fish boats, big and small. When I got home three hours later, I reflected back on all the strangers who had helped make it a nice trip. The woman who got up from her seat and reached out a hand to help me into the boat (a simple thing, but much appreciated), the couple who walked me back up the wharf after our little boat tour (a simple thing, but …), the boys who went to get me an ice cream while I sat in the car when my legs gave out (a simple thing, but …), the young woman who offered me a hand over the cement marker in the parking lot (a . . .) and finally the man in the line when I stopped to buy berries on the way home – he let me in front of him, when he saw I was 'on my last legs.'

It is wonderful to experience all that kindness, and I was glad I had gone on my own; I could have missed all of it. If you never need them, you never know how helpful and good-hearted people can be.

Now, lest this all be too tinted by rose-coloured glasses, I should balance it by saying the key to me is whether or not I really need help. People making assumptions about what I need, getting off on being a rescuer, are a problem.

On that trip to look at the river, people who helped me were all in synch with my desire for help – that brought tears to my eyes on more than one occasion (OK, OK, that means nothing, just a bit of MSy MenopauSal sentimentality).

Do you ever wonder what people see when they see you with your walker or chair or cane? I worry that the image I present is either needier than I really am, usually when I'm using the scooter, or not as needy, using the cane, having to balance, with tons of discomfort. Do my eyes and the set of my mouth tell them? Should I wear a sign with switchable plates: Neediness Index: extreme, moderate, low? Or should I have taken down the addresses of those people by the river and just gone to live with them?

LETTING GO

Of all the symptoms of MS we can talk about, the one which you may find most difficult to read and think about is bladder and bowel problems. The ol' neurogenic bladder – well trained but undependable, moody, capricious. "The waterworks." "The plumbing." We have various euphemisms which betray our discomfort with the whole topic of elimination. So here's where you should stop if seeing the words "accident", "pee" or "catheter" makes you wish you'd opted for a video instead of a book today.

People with MS were all once put-off by the topic. But like every one of the challenges with MS, familiarity with this one breeds – well, it breeds familiarity. I've dealt with both bowel and bladder accidents so often I can't help but feel familiar with them. Turns out, it's not all that bad, once I got my head around the idea that I had to deal with, cope with something which brought back only childish language and guidelines. And there are ways to cope with obnoxious waterworks or rebellious bowels. The best news has been that as my coping skills increased, the problem decreased. Our discussion here begins with conversations Flora and I had starting in 1998. And this is one of the areas where there's been change for the better since then.

Linda to Flora:

I am glad you got over that flare-up so quickly and that you are going to try to prevent another through better bladder management. Who would have thought peeing could be so darned complicated, eh? As promised, I'm gong to list for you all the things I am doing or have done to prevent infection and increase bladder control. There was a period five or more years ago when I was having infections, followed by antibiotics, all too often, three or four times a year at the worst.

At this point, I very rarely have accidents as I used to so often and I have not had an infection for years. Although I still have a neurogenic bladder, I feel as if I am controlling it. Various things that have helped are:

Cranberry juice, at least half a cup every morning.

Mandelamine, a drug that I now take only when I suspect the start of an infection. Like cranberry juice, it acidifies the urine. Originally, I used to take it every day to raise the pH level of my urine. It also acted as a gentle antiseptic, my pharmacist says. He also tells me it's seldom used now (I'm starting to feel old!), and doctors prescribe a low dosage of antibiotic (Bactrim) to be taken every day instead. Mandelamine was prescribed for me by a urologist – have you seen one? I had a cystoscopy, and a horrid extensive bladder testing session, the name of which escapes me. All of which confirmed that yes, I did indeed have a neurogenic bladder. Duh!

Intermittent catheterization. This has had the most dramatic effect, since it allows my bladder to completely empty, which was the problem before. I use a catheter every two to three hours when I'm at home. When I'm out, I seldom use one, although I do always carry one in case I feel uncomfortable and want to fully empty. It was a shock when it was first suggested I should use catheters, but they turned out to be easy to use, and no more fuss than my reading glasses. And I do appreciate being antibiotic-free!

Flushing. I have in the past done this when I felt an infection starting. It was suggested to me, I think, by my GP. I simply drink as much fluid as I possibly can, and then urinate a lot, of course. This means I did little else but drink and pee for a morning and afternoon. I drank mostly cranberry juice and tea. It worked very well, but required free time to devote to it.

Ditropan, a common antispasmodic drug used for urinary tract. I took this daily for a while, and it helped reduce the frequency. Before I used catheters, however, I would feel the need to urinate but not be able to, in other words, an uncomfortable feeling.

Plantain, a common plant and herbal remedy that works much the same as Ditropan. At first I picked it in my local park, washed and boiled it. Later I bought it in dried form and made tea.

Acupuncture. I get treatments every week, and that always includes at least one needle for the bladder (inserted on the abdomen). When this was first begun several years ago, I noticed improvement in bladder control very quickly.

Mental discipline. I have had some success with training my bladder to hold more urine; when I'm at home, I tolerate the feeling of discomfort for longer and longer periods, so that gradually I am able to urinate less frequently without the discomfort. There are also physical exercises you can do, exercising the muscle by stopping and starting the flow.

Emotional state. Staying calm is crucial, I find. My bladder is my thermometer; it tells me quicker than anything when I'm stressed, even when I don't otherwise realize it. Maybe you've noticed that when you're talking to a particular person on the phone, you always feel like you need to urinate? I know that the more at peace I am, the quieter my bladder is. But that's true for just about every symptom of this disease.

Hydrotherapy. The coldest possible water on the pelvic area following a warm shower. I've been told that helps build muscle strength; it's free and doesn't take long, so why not? You do that too, don't you?

My bladder now doesn't give me much trouble, although I still urinate more frequently than most. I get up once during the night sometimes. But I have found no way to reduce the incontinence I suffer in connection with menstruation. It's usually one day, at the beginning of my period, and was one of the little challenges brought on by menopause. Middle-aged, Menopausal and MS – the triple Emmy!

Well, that's the full catalogue. I hope you find what will work for you.

Flora to Linda:

As you know, I have always had a lot of questions about this bladder thing. Why not? It impacts every day and every trip out of the house. Your experiences are very helpful to hear about and, even though mine are different, they aren't that varied. I certainly agree about cranberry and am trying out the concentrate form daily as well as some juice in the morning. Cranberry juice sounds so available when in fact of course, it must be pure (and sour!) juice, not the usual cocktail stuff which is always laced with sugar. A question about daily incontinence – mostly dampness in fact. Incontinence sounds rather drastic. I find it more reassuring to wear a sanitary pad. Do you? I wonder what men do, not being set up for any monthly occurrences.

The hydrotherapy idea is interesting though I'm not sure I could take cold water.

Linda to Flora:

What I never understood was why no one ever explained the "MS bladder" to me, even after they discovered my bladder was not emptying fully, thus, infections. And why didn't they suggest catheters right away? I had to go through many infections and many treatments of antibiotics before an urologist suggested I learn to use catheters. Since then, I have no problem with infections. I know at the time it was a shock to have to use a catheter, but a little understanding of the emotional impact on the part of the urologist would have helped. The person who helped the most was the nurse from the Health

Unit; they're used to teaching home procedures, not the sterile clinical setting hospital nurses deal with. And the whole atmosphere of a nurse visiting me in my home and discussing the situation makes it a very comfortable relaxed encounter. Yea for Health Units!!

This may be far more than you care to know about bladders, my bladder in particular. I didn't realize what a long history of bladder stories I had, actually, until I started to think back. For a while, it was the most troublesome symptom and the constant use of drugs exacerbated my feeling of helplessness. That was back in the bad ol' days of my life with MS. I hope for you too this will soon be an episode from the bad ol' days!

Post Script:
Progress update: I have trained my bladder to not pester me for three hours, so my schedule does not revolve around bathroom visits. The training consisted of not heeding the first call for attention and gradually working the time up, first to 90 minutes, then 120, 150 and now 180. I also seldom have to get up during the night now.

You're probably not surprised to learn that Julie had her own contribution to this topic. Be warned – there's more – all three of us have done graduate level studies on the topic of elimination. And talk about it freely!

Julie to Linda:

Well here I am, armed and ready to discuss the two things to occupy my mind whenever planning a venture away from home. It doesn't matter how short the journey or inconsequential its purpose, the potential for disaster runs across my mind's eye like the stock quotations on Wall Street. The fickle bladder syndrome or much worse in my estimation, the volatile bowel situations that can develop in the span of a single breath are most unpleasant!! They are the two most difficult things to contend with when I think about the changes in my life caused by this testy little disease called MS. One event of "explosiveness" can reduce the dignity we struggle for to almost zip in a moments' notice. Talk about the ultimate feeling of no control over your life, a session with "Ms. Cranky Bowel" can cause several hours to several days of self-esteem recovery. When I think of the changes in my life that MS has caused, these are the ones that have given me moments of pure anguish. It has taken me a few years, to actually find methods to minimize and often even prevent those ugly moments. I've learned to take better care of myself, to eat right, to dress properly, to always know where the restroom is and make sure it's not up or down a flight of stairs, to make prophylactic" stops when traveling at about two to two and a half hour intervals, and most of all to expand my sense of humor. The sense of humor thing is so-o-o very important. If you take yourself too seriously, MS'll get you for sure. We can't always control what happens, but we're totally responsible for how we react to those situations. I guess "clean up and get on with what you're doing" is better than "find a corner to cry in." I've tried both and that second one can really wear you down. In regard to the bladder issue, this is what I've experienced.

I am fortunate in that I have never had a bladder infection associated with MS. I had one when I was in my twenties (a l-o-o-ng time ago), and that was almost thirty years before my diagnosis, so I think it's safe to say that there was no relation-ship. I have not had to self-catheterize yet, and seem to have no problem emptying. Gravity does a nice job for me with the addition of some pressure with the palm of my hand over the bladder area on my abdomen. The biggest problem I have is the spontaneous contraction of bladder muscle that causes an urgent need to pee "NOW!" I struggled with this for the first few years leading up to and after diagnosis. Shortly after my diagnosis, I saw a urologist, and had the usual bladder work-up, including a Cystometrogram. My neurogenic bladder was described to me as "an urge to empty at a lower than normal volume". I took Probanthene for about three years, and that helped a lot.

The urologist put me on Ditropan XL about a year ago, and I must say, the problem now isn't really a problem at all. I take 15mg. once a day, and function almost like normal. I do wear a pad if I think I may be away from appropriate facilities for an extended period, like when traveling and dealing with the unknown). I get up to go to the bathroom, usually once during the night. I don't consider that abnormal, and it hardly disturbs my sleep. I do find that once I know that I need a rest-room, it is very difficult for me to hold on and walk very far. Once my legs start to move, it's like pump action or some-thing. I don't like to have to concentrate on moving legs and controlling bladder at the same time.

Now for the really ugly issue for me. It is with no question the Academy Award winner in regard to dramatic effect. Though I seldom have a problem now because I am usually prepared, I was terrified that I would embarrass myself early on when I didn't understand what was happening. Unfortunately, the terror came true on a number of occasions, and I blamed every possible circumstance for the episodes, except the fact that my bowel was responding to confusing neural signals just like several other parts of my body. I have come to realize that it (poor thing) doesn't know when it's supposed to do what, so I try very, very hard to assist it in remembering. I drink a lot of water, because I'm totally convinced that helps keep thing from clogging up.

I eat a lot of fiber, snack on green peppers, celery, carrots, all kinds of fruit, etc., etc., etc. If we're going to be traveling, I add some Metamucil (Psyllium seeds) to my daily routine, just to make sure that if I don't access enough veggies & fruit, I'm covering that base anyway. I try to eat meals at regular times, because sometimes it's so tempting not to. I find that messes my system up totally. I use suppositories (glycerin) if I'm going to be out for an extended time, just to inspire some action and emptying before I'm away from familiar facilities. On those occasions where my schedule is really abnormal, and I feel as though I need some extra preparation, I use a Fleets enema to prepare. I don't know that I've ever been able to identify triggers for bouts of incontinent bowel. I think fat content of a meal has a role for me as it does for Flora, but I've never been sure of that. A couple of times that I had serious problems followed the ingestion of a big meal (both with steak, which I love rare, by the way), and one time when I had eaten a wonderful triple-dip monster ice cream cone.

Linda, when you say that these issues are difficult to talk about, you aren't just kidding. I even had trouble talking about the incontinent bowel with my Neurologist and my Internist. I worked with both of them at the hospital. They are both friends, and frankly, I was too embarrassed, even with my extensive background in healthcare, to describe it as it really was.

When asked if I had bowel problems, I said, "Occasional diarrhea", and of course they said that's not likely to be related to MS. Since I almost never suffer from constipation, which many MSers do, they felt that my bowel function was normal. I've had those awful moments in an airport, a restaurant on more than a couple of occasions, a shopping mall, several times while traveling (o-o-h it's a long way to a rest area when you have to go NOW), once during a birthday party in a big hall (with a bathroom down a flight of stairs), in Germany (twice). In the past two years, however, I have been so much better in this troubling area. It's only seven years since diagnosis, and I feel that in that time, I have learned so much about the management of this tricky disorder. We do become (M)a(S)ters of management, don't we?

Linda to Flora:

Can you stand a gruesome tale today? I hope so because I really need to tell someone, to get this off my chest. I'm in shock.

This morning I planned to go out to buy a few things at a drug store I drive to. (There's one I scooter to and one I drive to.) Had my breakfast and cleared my bowels, so I thought I was all set. Sashi (my dog) was excited as always by the thought of a trip in the car. But we made it only as far as the elevator when I thought I'd better go back and use the bathroom once more, just to be safe. Sashi was a little confused, but happy when we were once again on our way in just a few minutes. But again, those few steps, twenty yards, to the elevator were enough to jiggle my insides around, and I once again had to return to the apartment. At this point I was getting just a bit confused and worried. Why was this happening? I hadn't eaten anything different that I could think of. Should I just stay home this morning? Damn, damn, damn!

After the trip to the bathroom, I decided to press on, as I felt OK and generally hate to be alarmist or dramatically frightened of an accident. (Why, by the way, do we call loss of bowel control an accident?? It's no more an accident than a nosebleed is an accident.) This trip started out well – down to the elevator, wait for it to come, then ride down to parking. But as I walked over to my car, real trouble in my guts. I headed straight back to the apartment, (Sashi still in tow of course), but didn't make it. I just couldn't control it those last few steps, and the accident took place. This had happened a lot in the past, but not lately. I know it's nothing I have control over, I knew I'd been cautious this morning. So why? I was left with the usual feeling of impatience at the inconvenience of it all, the lengthy bathroom work to clean up. And that all takes energy, which I'd rather spend elsewhere, as you might guess.

I got angry at the power MS was trying to exert over me, and determined not to let it rule my life, at least not this morning. So I went off to the store, a little tired and none too cheery. I was making a point, but for whom?

Sashi was, of course, very happy when she was finally able to take her place in the back seat, surveying the cars and world around us like an imperious landlord. When we got back home, I noticed for the first time, her way of telling me she had not dealt patiently with all the false starts – she had dragged bathroom garbage under the bed and tore it to shreds.

I don't know if I'll send this, but it sure feels better to talk it through. I still have no idea what upset my bowels today, though. Do you ever have this problem? Please tell me that you used to but have found a simple way to avoid it.

Flora to Linda:

Unfortunately I have to second the motion. And yesterday would you believe. Both events were part of my use of oil, the first time olive oil and this time flax oil.

The trigger event is amount of oil. A little each day is controllable but not quite enough for daily bowel movements. I went to twice a day (seemed to make sense) but it led to an out of control situation. Not diarrhea. So I am back to oil once a day (or will be) and long earnest sessions on the toilet. The effects for us both seem very different so I have no good information except that it's – guess what – MS.

Thanks for hanging in there with us. It's a topic we just can't talk to many people about. "How am I? Got a leaky bladder and no bowel control, but otherwise, just hunky-dory, how are you?" I really, really appreciate having MS pals I can talk to openly and even laugh with about this.

DEALING WITH BLOOD

Whether we like it or not, no person is an island. We are born into a family; they are with us 'til death us do part; then there's the family we choose or create, our spouse and children. Families are together in sickness and in health. So if one in the family has a disease, the whole family is implicated. And for someone with MS, it can prove just as difficult to deal with the reaction of family members to the disease and changed reality as it is to deal with their own. For better or worse, family is very important in determining how someone with MS copes, and the impact the disease has on their quality of life. But what a test illness is for relationships; marriages can break down under the weight, cracks in relationships can become gullies. Often ill health is even hard to talk about.

But small children have none of that – they often think wheelchairs and scooters are fun, and a cane a wonderful prop . They don't know that these things are in any way a problem. Flora and Julie take great delight in their grandchildren and I in reading about them. Our talk of adult family relationships gets more serious, of course.

Flora to Linda:

My daughter Sarah will be here this month as well, with her daughter. Did you know that my two grandchildren were born three weeks apart, both in the same month in 1998? I will confess to some bad moments realizing I was not going to be that sort of grandmother I had always thought. But the books I have sent are pretty well ones I know by heart, and we can play on the beach, if not walk on the beach, and soon, when they are up to speed which won't be far off from the looks of things, I can send them both e-mail messages for a parent to read to them. We talk on the phone – more or less – and I will learn to say "Hi" in Swedish and even in New Yorkese. A number of the grandparent style adaptations I work on have as much, maybe more, to do with distance as disability.

My children and I talked about the genetic aspects of MS early on. Their concern about the disease was all from my perspective; for some reason I haven't worried about them or the babies. Maybe that prospect is just unthinkable for me.

At this point, my kids are more optimistic about medical science and its proposed therapies than I am. Though, yes, I am still on Betaseron injections every second day, and no, nothing startling and wonderful has yet happened. On the other hand, I have had no attacks this winter and my energy and spirits remain high.

Linda to Flora:

I must admit a bias on my part; since I am single without kids, I am really curious about how those with a spouse and/or kids deal with MS.

When you speak of PwMS, are you thinking of flesh and blood types or the myriad of people we meet on the Internet, through the newsgroups? I have found the latter to be rather frustrating, as I cannot remember one from the other enough to follow anyone's progress. I made notes at one point on what I knew about this one and that one, but I have never had the patience to go check those notes before I read their latest message. I really value people like you who I talk to or e-mail on a regular basis, good days as well as bad. I get a sense of what your and their life is like and what they have to cope with. I trust what they say to me as reality as they see it, not an ego-trip or a competitive game. But maybe you're talking about them too, those people we get to know personally.

They're the only people, I feel, who really understand what living with this disease is like. Others, family or friends, try very hard but have no reference point to help them really know what it's like. They've been tired lots of times, but they've never had nerve fiber fatigue. They've lost their balance, but they don't have a problem with balance. Etc., etc. Still, I really appreciate those who listen and who try to get a grasp of this thing called MS as it relates to me. I wish I had the energy to talk more about it when the time is right; I wish my mind worked quickly enough to respond when there is what teachers call a teachable moment.

Have you ever gone to a self-help group? I went a few times many moons ago, but at the time was not ready to be sitting around with other people who were in worse shape than I was.

I had to get to a point of acceptance, I think, before that was possible or helpful. I do know that many people find a lot of support that way.

Someone on the newsgroup just posted a message about dealing with children when you have MS. Did you read it? I'm sure he's not alone in having worried about how his kids, aged nine and twelve, would deal with a father, formerly very active, who now could not participate. The good news is he reports that his girls are more mature as a result of the disease in the family and having more responsibility, e.g., shopping and paying for groceries, which he can no longer do. He's still there in the most important way, to talk and especially listen. I've heard people say that in that regard, PwMS may have an advantage, those who are more homebound than they would otherwise be. They spend much more time actually talking to their kids. This appeals to the teacher in me and as an MSer, I'm always glad to hear the bright side of the situation.

I've seen people with illness try to hide it from the kids, who were pre-teens, old enough to have some level of understanding, and I wonder if that isn't a bit patronizing, as well as denying them the chance to learn very important lessons they will need someday themselves, how to deal with illness, having a responsible attitude toward their own body and health. It also denies them the chance to participate, to help, to have a responsible role. What think you? You're a parent, so I'm anxious to know how you see it, even though your kids were adults when you were diagnosed.

Julie and I were to meet face-to-face when I went back to Ontario to visit family. It turns out that she's really only three or four hours away from Stratford, where I went to visit my mother. As we talked about meeting, I realized that I knew about her family, the people in her life – husband, daughters and grandkids, but had told her nothing of my family members. I wrote, and rewrote and rewrote a message to her to fill her in, and felt as if I was doing my own cognitive therapy session. It's tough to describe family dynamics to someone who doesn't know all the people involved, and very difficult to keep perspective. It would be unfair to just whine, hence the rewriting of the message. My family knows little about my life with MS; I talk regularly to only one sister, and then seldom about MS. I'm as much a factor in the family chemistry, or lack of, as anyone, I know. I understand rationally some of the factors that are at play but still there's a sense of sorrow and regret.

Linda to Julie:

I haven't told you much about my family. We're stoic, dutiful, hard-working, conscientious, and weak on communication. I have lived on this side of the Rockies, over 3,000 miles away for almost thirty years; it's a distance we can't seem to deal with easily. When I do see family members, my mother, a brother, and two sisters, we never talk about MS; I don't volunteer information and they don't ask. The need for backbone is a common theme, voiced or implied. Illness is a failing, somehow, maybe even shameful?

But we don't really communicate on an intimate level about any personal challenges. It was hard in the bad years to not feel support behind me, but my younger sister now regularly provides material support, doing what she can, and more importantly, she expresses a desire to keep in touch. Meanwhile I've developed into the independent cuss I am. And am better able to cope on my own than I might have been. I believe there's a unity to our lives, that the pieces do all fit together. We fashion and are fashioned by our experiences; we develop the skills and strategies we need. I'm strong-willed and independent because I've had to be. My mother would probably say the same thing about herself. In the end I'm not sure it's harder to have a family who never talks about their individual stuggles, than the other extreme. In my family not paying too much attention may be a vote of confidence?

My father had MS, and I, as well, took it all too casually. I didn't ask questions, or keep close track of how he was doing. Why not? I ask myself now. It's the biggest regret of my life. Dad died twenty years ago; I was in the middle of my first MS attack at the time, but didn't know for another year and a half that's what it was.

All of this comes up when I think of going home, which I do every year or so. This trip I will see Mom, who is turning eighty-four, but is still quite well, and Susan, my younger sister. I get a little stressed out around family, but I'm going to stay off the coffee and overdose on Chamomile so I'll be palatable.

Boy, this all got kinda heavy, eh? I think I need to go out for a break. But it is so nice to share with you, Julie.

Linda L. Ironside

Julie to Linda:

Families are all so different, aren't they? I mean to say that we all have roots, and it's funny sometimes to think about how we become who we are. Some parts of our personalities are because of our family's influence, and some things develop because we fight that influence or kind of in spite of it. You know what I mean? I don't know how I would handle not being able to talk to family about what I'm experiencing. Yet, sometimes the best and most meaningful and comforting conversations are with someone totally unrelated, and yet who has a sincere interest, like our cyber-conversations have been.

Anyway, it would be nice if your Mom could view your MS as a part of your life that she wanted to understand. I think it tends to be a bit of a generational issue. My mother died of Breast Cancer in 1970. The entire time she was ill, neither of my parents ever used the word "cancer" to each other or to my brother or I. That was a span of almost three years. I knew, because I worked in health care then too and knew the stages she was going through and certainly recognized the drugs they were using. It amazes me to this day that so many difficult moments could have been avoided and those last few months especially could have been more peaceful for her if she could have just brought all of the things in her mind to closure before she died. I kind of think she did, but I don't think the rest of us ever did really. My dad would not let the doctors discuss anything with my brother or I. Heck, we were well beyond being children, but that was intended to protect us. It also was intended to prevent anything from interrupting that stoic style of dealing with illness that you describe in your family. I kind of recognize what you describe. My Mom would have been eighty-five this year, so we are talking about people of the same period.

Mine is one of those families which has multiple cases of Multiple you-know-what. A cousin has it. My father had it. And I have felt closer to him since my diagnosis than I ever did before. I have found something very personal we share. But too late for me to try to understand what he was going through, for us to talk about our shared challenge. But not too late for me to carry out a promise I made when he died – to give voice to his sense of humour and carry on his love of laughter. Though I didn't know then just how badly I would need that nor how hard it might be.

Linda to Julie:

Thursday. My father died twenty years ago today, and I am honouring him by talking to people about him. And maybe trying to expunge the guilt I feel about my lack of support when he was alive. Do you remember that he had MS? We, the family took it all very much in stride, as we did any of life's curve balls. I lived on the other side of the country but wasn't phoning, writing, connecting.

My MS diagnosis has connected me, all right. It's full of irony – that, of the four kids, I'm the one who carries on with MS, the one probably least close to Dad. Is there some Karma at work here? That I also was given his sense of humour (though my memory's not as good), which is a great help. That he died during my first attack. That his death meant I didn't get into hospital for tests . . . so was not diagnosed . . . so went off to China as planned . . . so became who I am now. And I would have become someone different if he had died later or earlier.

Linda L. Ironside

Christmas! A time for families, yes, but also for friends.
For excess, for power socializing no matter if you're with
family or not. Also a time when desires far outreach
possibility for PwMS. As is the case with just about
everyone else as well, to be sure. We're not all that differ-
ent, we just get that "Xmas glaze" look and bow out a
little sooner than others our age.

Julie to Linda:

Haven't heard from you in a while, it must be Christmas. My
goodness, the last two weeks have been busy. It's funny when I
say that, because my definition of busy is so different from
what it used to be. Because we travel a little bit right after
Christmas, I'm kind of getting ready to be away for a few days
(Tennessee till January 2nd). I have such a good time buying
gifts and yet, such a hard time, both of which were wonderful
days, but quite taxing in terms of energy and focus for a few
days afterward. Oh, I guess there's a price to pay for the
wonderful things. They are things that I can't imagine doing
without. I also have had some very nice get-togethers with
friends. Dinner out or visits at their or my home. All in all, this
has been a most unusual holiday season. We Zubys normally
lead a fairly quiet existence and we love it that way. Michael
and I spent the day yesterday wrapping grandchildren things. I
love doing that, and can handle anything that's relatively
small. Most of what we're giving them is little stuff, but some
exceeded my capacity for handling. Mike can wrap a pretty mean
package, and did several things for me. Well, enough of that!

I'm actually having a great time getting ready for this
Christmas. I'm just so tired, that in a way, I'm looking forward

to a few days of just being in sit-in-the-car-and-travel mode. When we go down to Tennessee, we visit with a family, originally from Michigan who is like an extension of our own. Michael and Gary grew up together and have always been very close. One of their children is a goddaughter and her birthday celebration will be on Sunday. Other than that, I don't expect any hoopla. Should be a pretty quiet week.

I sincerely hope that the holidays give you an opportunity to focus on the life that you've developed in BC, that the friendships you've kindled in those many years provide strength and give value to the season. I, like you, don't affiliate with any practice of religion – I think of the Christmas season, myself, as a time to focus on the little ones, but as you might imagine, I do get rather philosophical during the holidays. My growing years were in the Lutheran Church and Mike's in the Catholic. We sort of raised our children to make choices in terms of practice, for themselves, but didn't direct them to any particular faith. I suppose that in terms of belief, mine centers somewhere around a Luthero-Catholic (made that up) core. Having no affiliation now though doesn't take away the fact that there are deep-rooted values in our lives. I think that we are very spiritual people, but don't align ourselves with any particular formal practice. And, actually, I think that's not a bad thing.

MS is, as they say, a family affair, as is any serious illness. Everyone is tested, everyone must make adjustments, must find the very deepest level of their relationship. The world gets all topsy-turvy; natural caregivers must learn to accept rather than give help, children learn how to help Mom or Dad, siblings come to know that they cannot rely as they may once have done on the rock of the family. And lovers learn new ways of both measuring and expressing love.

Julie to Linda:

Mike bought me a great thermal cup with lid that I navigate with, so that we don't have to buy new carpeting every few months. Mike works hard enough all day and then yardwork, etc., so I hate to leave silly household chores for him too. If something needs to be lifted or moved or something like that, I save it for him. He'd very readily do it·all, but that would be awfully unfair.

My daughters both have lovely families and could easily use a break once in a while. There's a place where I wish I could be of help and just step in for a day, but I just can't. In terms of my wonderful partner of thirty-six years now, there can't be another guy like him, and I feel very fortunate. We have always had a strong relationship with a lot of love as well as true friendship. The most difficult thing I deal with, pertaining to MS, is what I know that it has done to him. Obviously, by virtue simply of age, we're not the frisky pair that we used to be. But the effects of spasticity, nonfunctional or erratically functional body parts adds new meaning to the word "challenge." We have no problem expressing our love to each other, verbally or physically, and I hope to heck that we'll always be able to do that.

You made a statement that is so true: That each of us fashions a life that suits us!

Linda to Julie:

Good to realize that it's what you do about what happens to you that steers you forward. Sounds like you've both taken this in stride, as you have so many of the new challenges in your life. People have complained that the MS Society doesn't offer much help dealing with intimacy and MS. Have you found any materials which could be a support?

Better let Mike know I'm putting together a proposal for the MS society to clone him, as one solution for others. Just as this disease tests us as individuals, it is also a test of the strength of a relationship, I guess, as is surely any crisis you have to face together. Or what?

Me, I'm on the other end, not only living alone, but not even interested in romance. Less and less. Is that MS? I think sometimes I am so busy living so as to minimize the effects of MS, there's not much room for romance. There's an irony, eh? It's a disease that makes bed one of my favourite places to be but also takes away the desire to make full use of it. I'm tired even thinking of it. I'm gonna go lie down.

Julie to Linda:

With regard to MS Society assistance on intimacy issues, I never really went looking there, but they have such a big library of resource materials, it would seem like that important topic would be high on the list. We have sort of come to grips with the fact that traditional moves and dexterity aren't feasible . . . creativity reigns . . . communication, such a difficult thing for any of us to do at the right time and in the right way, but so-o-o important. Yes, I would probably consent to the cloning of my husband, but I would definitely keep the original Michael.

One of my greatest concerns regarding Michael and my MS pertains to the scope of the impact that my physical changes have had on his need to be the primary doer of thing that I used to handle. Even more though, I worry about the disappointment he must feel in regard to what we had planned to do in our future. Just my lack of flexibility and adaptability limits where we can go and what we can do. If it doesn't stop us totally, it certainly causes us to think about how. Those are things that I think about a lot, and though he doesn't often verbalize them, I'm sure he does too. I often think about how I have been able to learn to deal with my MS, and much of the credit for that goes to him. He is a wonderful reason for me to want to, as are my daughters and their families. But none of them deserve having to deal with my MS. It is a burden that, particularly for Mike, seems so unfair and creates changes in his life that will make it additionally hard for him as he faces changes in himself (age and health related), due to my limitations.

Incidentally, my mother-in-law is eighty-four years old and beginning to have some health problems, needing oxygen at times in order to remain somewhat active. We spend a lot of summer weekends with her at Hubbard Lake, and the dear lady will see me struggling up the porch steps or maneuvering something through the house, and literally throw herself in front of me to intervene. Part of my reaction is frankly declining the offer of help and then feeling guilty because I probably hurt her feelings. She's a wonderful person and a very nurturing personality. Part of my reaction stems from the fact that I feel as though I should care for her (fifty-eight yrs vs. eighty-one and all), and that makes me feel *so* inadequate. She told me a few months ago that Michael told her to let me do things my way, and to follow his cues. He just seems to know when to step in, and she really has controlled her urge to take care of me admirably, so guess that means that he's a good teacher. She's stopped leaping in front of me, and we laugh about it now, but it was a real issue for me for a long time. I just didn't know how to tell her to stop hovering over me or gasping when I tripped, etc. She's a great lady and I'm so lucky to have her. She also raised a pretty wonderful son, and I love her dearly for giving me that.

I decided to ask Julie's husband for some feedback, just to get his perspective. Here's what he wrote:

Michael to Linda:

Julie tends to overreact to what she thinks might upset, bother, or frustrate me. So I'm careful not to say anything that might make her try to compensate.

I don't think I had much of a conscious reaction to her diagnosis, other than to try and support her. She seems to cope with MS quite well. Thank God she has a very upbeat attitude towards things in general.

That being said, I was not very happy at work around the time of her diagnosis. My present employer came along and made me an offer that I couldn't refuse, so I didn't. Looking back at it, I now believe the anger at work was actually because of Julie's affliction. It was just something that I needed time to adjust to.

Presently, I seem to have accepted where we are and what may or may not happen to us in the future. We need to make the best of everything while we can and just hope that the MS progresses slowly.

In order to cope, you must first be able to realize that you have to make adjustments to your own head. You've got to be able to realize who you are and where you're going, and then refocus your perspective. Everyone is in control of their own destiny.

Everyone has a family though they're not always blood relations. The people who support us, who listen when things get tough, who laugh with us. Self-help groups can become family in all the important ways. As can the friends who follow the low and high tides of our lives by phone or e-mail. Some people live on the mainland, but some, though they may be islands, are part of a large archipelago.

Writing a book about MS would be a lot easier if I didn't have MS, I once told a friend. I explained the irony behind that line, that MS provides the material, but also gives me problems with concentration, memory, manual dexterity, and fatigue, which all interfere at times with this project. MS has often slowed down work on this book, but seldom stopped it altogether, as it did when I was confronted with a brand new and temporarily very disabling symptom.

Linda L. Ironside

STOP THE PRESSES!!

It's January, 2000 and the start of a new millennium. The manuscript is almost finished – great! Y2K didn't happen – great! No big health problems, just too much tension – great?

But in bed, 10 p.m. my face was struck with lightning, again and again, here, there, all over the left side. I cried in pain for a couple hours, thinking this must be the facial pain I had heard mentioned. What should I do?

This was the start of my next MS chapter, a new kind of attack for me, Trigeminal Neuralgia (TGN or TN). The start of a period of confusion, fear, anxiety, continual emotional pain which overlay the occasional physical. As with most MS exacerbations, it radically altered my life. I cancelled every outing, every appointment. My fear took the shape of familiar questions. What was going to happen to me? Was this the way the MS was going to get me in the end? Would I ever drive again, use my walker outdoors, tutor the boys, finish the book? Would I ever stop crying? (How many MS attacks do I have to have before each one will not elicit the fear that it is forever, I now wonder.) Where was the cheery optimism I was so proud of? Was I a fraud?

My life had fallen apart, and I was in full panic mode. I couldn't put it in any kind of perspective, and was really surprised at the answer when someone asked how long I'd been on the drug which only added to my grief, though it did control the pain. It had been only four days! The nurse/saint I talked to assured me my body would adjust to it and I would feel better, which turned out, of course, to be the case. I could smile again.

So, with Tegretol controlling the TGN, I'm back at it, it being the life I enjoyed just three weeks ago. Of course, I had shared my pain, my terror, with my friends who would understand.

Linda to Julie:

No fair!! I seem to be the only one having Y2K electrical glitches, and they're in my face! Trigeminal Neuralgia – sounds sort of catholic, doesn't it? My introduction to MS pain, although it feels as if I've moved right ahead to the graduate level. It started, out of the blue, a week ago, sudden jabs of pain, spasms, whenever I moved a muscle on the left side of my face. I had one day of not eating and barely talking. Crying, which is a rather instinctive response to pain, it seems, made everything worse, which I found particularly cruel. I got on Baclofen and things calmed down for a while, with spasms invading only very periodically. Until this morning, when I had another spell of a couple hours, even though I had tried to appease the beast with the drug. And I'm so tired, one of the effects of TGN, I'm told.

Now that I have your attention, let me continue my tale of MS woe. I lost a big flap of dead skin off my foot this week. Ouch! Skin, it turns out, is rather nicer to walk on than bare flesh. MS-related – poor circulation. No drug for this one, so I cancelled everything on my schedule for the week and moved to survival mode. Friends helped get me to the doctor, change the dressing on my foot, keep the cupboards stocked and me sane. The GP who looked at my foot, not my regular, was obviously in the mood for something a little more medically interesting, and said nothing about circulation nor the fact that this can turn into something serious.

The most critical in this network of caregivers has been, I think, a friend who has MS with whom I spoke on the phone every day. Dee Dee is also dealing with acute MS right now, so we have lots to share. But what's been special for me is that she can still laugh, in fact, likes to laugh. Some of our jokes are pretty gruesome, but we enjoy them.

Then today someone phoned to let me know the Annette Funicello story, the Hollywood B-movie actress stricken with MS, was on TV. I watched only a few minutes before I came to my senses and realized this was not the time for this kind of entertainment.

So, after twenty-three years, I finally have experience with MS pain, the physical kind. It's been difficult to learn that the pain of spasms is ... spasmodic. When I had a few hours without spasms, I tended to think this little MS chapter was over, and then was thrown into despair when it was back. Everyone with MS has dealt with the terrible uncertainty of it all, the lack of dependable prognosis or even treatment. That is, I think, the lesson for me to learn from this. To accept that this is happening, to accept that it will take a while to figure out how best to deal with it, including the drug regimen, to *accept*. The pain would be lessened, I'm sure, if I weren't so shocked and insulted by it. It's only pain, after all, which is what I tell myself when I absolutely must brush my teeth.

My walking program, getting out each day for a walk down the street with my dog and my walker has been put on hold and I can already feel physical atrophy. But I'll soon be walking on skin again and will be out there practicing correct walking, as before. Maybe with more appreciation for the gift of walking.

I like to think through what's happening and my reaction to it, and am glad you're there, Julie, on the other end of my musings. Anything here to respond to? Don't feel obliged if there isn't. I'll be more than happy to read about reunion plans and grandkids and even weather.

Julie to Linda:

I'm hoping that you are doing better. I know a letter was promised for yesterday, and instead of writing, I went visiting at my daughter's house for the day. While I was there, I fell in the bathroom, hit my head on the bathtub, and am nursing a bump today. I just don't feel like looking at the computer screen for very long, so I'm stalling another day. Just didn't want you to think I'd forgotten.

Linda to Julie:

Can we agree not to do ourselves in at the same time? Your head hurts, my head hurts, gets a bit boring, doesn't it? And hitting your head on the tub sounds just a bit too dangerous. Let's keep these little "extreme adventures of the unhealthy kind" just a little less dramatic, shall we?

I expect you had more to deal with than a little bump and hope you're feeling all right now. How are your eyes? I guess I'll know that when you start visiting the computer again.

I thought the TGN was history, until this morning when it came back big time. Back to no eating and teeth brushing only between bouts. Luckily I had an appointment with the neurologist this afternoon, who said that Baclofen was not the drug of choice. Suddenly I felt like one of the privileged class when he put me on Tegretol. I took one right away and was a tad disappointed when two hours later, I couldn't safely open my mouth wider than to slip in a piece of paper (don't ask!). Got an attack while on the phone, which is a real conversation stopper.

My foot is almost healed, so as soon as I clear my head of drug effects, I can go walking again. Things *are* getting better!

I really hope you didn't do any serious damage, Julie. And will look forward to hearing from you when you're up to it. By the way, Happy Chinese New Year!

A couple of days later, I received the promised e-mail from Julie:

Julie to Linda:

Though at times I am for sure a pain in someone's butt, the kind of pain that I experience related to MS is pain in the back! I have never experienced what you are going through right now, Linda, the TGN, Trigeminal Neuralgia. It sounds positively awful, and I'm concerned about whether or not you are getting enough to eat and drink. You've been suffering with this for a while now. I remember when you and I met in Stratford, we enjoyed several meals together. If I recall accurately, you were careful to select foods that agreed with you and that you liked, but also food that covered the nutritional bases. That's almost impossible to do when the act of separating jaws only slightly results in awful pain. I know that my expression of concern won't make the pain go away, but perhaps it will help by making you feel a little emotional comfort.

Well, I'm going to describe my back pain in the same kind of terms that I've used when trying to tell a doctor about the way it feels. Long before I knew that I had MS, and certainly to the present time, I've had periods of severe back pain. These episodes usually last about three to four weeks, occur every few months, and are most horrific upon waking up in the morning. The pain generally subsides within an hour or so of arising, and after that the worst I experience for the rest of the day is a dull backache. The sensation I feel upon waking is like a knife cutting through my spinal cord. I am just certain that if I move in the wrong way, my upper body will separate from the lower and I'll never again have it all together – not that I'm very together at normal times – hee hee! The pain feels hot, searing, tearing, and other stuff like that. I've used those terms with my neurologist as well as my regular physician. They really can't comprehend what I'm talking about, and though they sincerely have tried to find the root cause (X-rays, etc.) neither of them thinks it is directly caused by MS, nothing has really ever shown up as the potential offender. I am absolutely convinced that it is part of my pattern of disease. I think that there is a certain amount of spasm in my back, and I think also that because there is weakness in spite of trying to compensate with exercise for back strength. Those episodes have coincided with exacerbations in recent years and I suspect that in the earlier years before I knew what was going on that they did too – about twice every year.

At these times, lifting and maneuvering myself into a sitting position on the edge of the bed when I first wake up results in excruciating pain. It brings tears to my eyes and causes my legs to totally stiffen up like rigid tree trunks. The only way I can get off the side of the bed is by very slow, deliberate, short movements, assisted by canes, a nearby closet door, or if my understanding husband is nearby, his loving support. I've given credit for some relief, to the early morning Baclofen that I take, and coupled with a couple of extra strength

Tylenol. At least I feel like I'm being proactive, even if they don't deserve credit for the pain subsiding. It does diminish within about one to one and a half hours even if I don't take anything, so I think that it is perhaps in part brought on by lying in one position for extended periods during the night . . . who knows!! It's just been one of those things that I like to try to explain to myself, but for which there is probably no logical single explanation. As with so many weird body things, it's just an MS thing. You know what I'm saying?

That's my pain-related input. I've been told that some people with MS have the sensation of a belt or a rope being tightened around their waist. Maybe this is my version of whatever causes the belt thing for some. I would prefer a belt or rope, but nobody asked for my preferences. Oh well!

Please take care of that jaw thing. I truly hope that it subsides soon, and that you spring back into your usual normal form again.

Reading about Julie's back pain made my own feel less overpowering. My bouts with TGN certainly have been the most dramatic chapter in my MS story. But my timing was good. I was connected to friends online so had lots of people to talk to during the time I was more or less panic-stricken and homebound.

MS – PUBLIC PERCEPTIONS

People the world over are enjoying the benefits of the new technology, the digital world. No one, perhaps, more than people with a disability, who can research their medical condition from home; they can shop for the latest in equipment and medical aids, and they can communicate with others around the globe about similar problems. Computers have reduced the handicaps in disability. They also reduce the psychological aspect, providing a very social life and a creative one for the 'talkers', those who like to write. And best of all, computers are fun! There really was no need to explain all this to Flora, but I did.

Linda to Flora:

How are you this week, Flora? Ready to hit the keyboard again? I was talking to a friend t'other day, who asked if cyberland is a great boon to me, in dealing with MS. It's wonderful how freely I can share MS experiences, even work on a book with someone I've never met. I appreciate being in contact with people at all levels of MS, which broadens my perspective on the disease. I also like being able to ask questions so quickly of the real MS practitioners, the people at the front lines. All in all, it's very lucky, I think, if you have MS, to be living in the high-tech age. I really can't imagine how lonely and isolated people must have been in the past. Especially since not everyone can get out to meetings of self-help groups. I know you don't use the voice activated programs, at least the ones I've read on the newsgroups. Have you ever thought of using them? Is there anything else to aid you? What kind of screen magnifier is available? What is needed, yet to be developed?

For me, sitting here in front of a screen is a very nice place to be; it's the place where MS has the least power in my life, and I can more or less forget about it, except for the too frequent bathroom trips. So I am very happy it's 1999, not 1969, and value what technology allows me to do. No way would I be sitting at my desk writing letters on a typewriter! I also enjoy belonging to MS newsgroups and read the mail every day. Do you? And what about MS web pages? Do you surf? I must admit I find the vast array of info. available all a little too technical for me, but I like being kept up to date as to the latest theories and treatments. I love things like Jooley's Joint, the cyber penpal service for PwMS. That's how I met Julie, you remember. This is all so new, I still am tickled by the idea of our correspondence and where it has led. I remember seeing my first tape recorder in elementary school and thinking I would some day like to have a gadget like that. And now we have the computer.

On the other hand, it still doesn't do diddlysquat about the heat, though, does it?

Why do people still gasp when I tell them I have MS? Why will people not talk about it, ask questions? Maybe they have a misconception of what the disease is, maybe they assume the worst, maybe that's (the worst case scenario) all they know. In fact, "I have MS" can mean everything from no visible signs to being completely bedridden. Because mobility is the most noticeable symptom, MS is often associated with a wheelchair as a given. It's often confused with Muscular Dystrophy. And

MS neurogenic fatigue is all too often seen as lack of will or discipline ("You should exercise more.").

Public education is badly needed. People with MS and the MS Society have a big job to do in educating people; it's not as bad as people think, but it may also be worse – not always a crippler but there can be a lot of symptoms which are invisible.

The English film, "Hilary and Jackie", was a red flag for me on the issue of public perception and I was glad to get Julie's more balanced perspective on it.

Linda to Julie:

Remember the movie, "Hilary and Jackie?" The one about the cellist, Jacqueline duPre, who had MS. I went to see it last week, although another friend who has MS told me not to – too depressing. I have read every review I could find and no one made much of the fact she had MS. I wish I could remember what you thought of it; I hope you'll remind me. My reaction was very strong; I found the film depressing, and very superficial in its treatment of the disease. I, like my friend, am concerned about the public image it presents; we have worked so long to update old stereotypes of MS – you'll be using a wheelchair soon, there's no medical intervention available, there's no hope.

The friend who first alerted me to problems with the film worries even more, that people who see the movie will think all people with MS become a bit crazy like Jackie, that sexual deviance is somehow part of it too. What do you think is the public perception of MS, and the possible effect of this film, now out on video, so available to a much greater audience? I think that public awareness is one of the biggest jobs of the MS Society, and they should try to counter the image this film portrays. Interesting that the movie review in our national paper, MS Canada, (April, 1999) as well as the one in the US magazine of the MS Society, (Inside MS, Spring 1999) does not touch on the potential impact on the public as far as awareness of MS goes.

The American reviewer did say, "The movie has a mix of misinformation and very realistic scenes about the disease." The reviewer also mentioned that the progression of her (Jackie's) disease seemed too rapid in the film, and was somewhat frightening. I think it's important that people learn that MS varies a great deal from person to person, that you really can't leap to conclusions for all of us with the disease. I've done my bit for public awareness – I wrote up something for the Vancouver Sun, but don't know if they will take it, of course.

Julie to Linda:

I didn't see it as a negative presentation at all, given what I think the purpose of the film was. Jackie's condition certainly was horrible, and for those who might be seeing it, having been newly diagnosed, I agree with you that it might be an awful experience. Since the movie's main objective, I think, however, was the relationship of the two sisters, and as you say, seen from Hillary's perspective, it attained that goal. I hope that the MS society hasn't made recommendations to people about the film's potential to educate about MS. That I think would be totally inappropriate, as you feel.

It does depict one form of the nasty little disease, but probably only six to nine per cent or so of the thousands of people who have it. That being said, if the other 91-94 per cent were told to see it, the risk of scaring the hell out of them should be a BIG concern and a total disservice to the MS community. We (Mike watched it too) thought that it was a very interesting story of H & J's relationship and the tensions that came about because of their incredible talents as well as the polar opposite directions that they chose for their lives. Each, we felt, had strong yearnings for the other's circumstances. The methods of coping were certainly dependent on each sister's personality. There was definitely a clear indication of several characteristics in their relationship: jealousy about the other's success in their chosen life path, dependency on the other for approval and dependency on the other to satisfy or fill a gap for their individual disappointments. We both thought that it was a pretty complicated story. There were four wet eyes in this house Sunday night, inasmuch as we did look at the potential for MS and feel some possible peek into the future, but also 'cause it was a sad story of sisters.

Linda to Julie:

My, what a wonderful review you wrote! You could market yourself as a film/video reviewer!

I agree with you about what the film was trying to do/say and not do/say. My concern is that since it received quite a lot of publicity, here at least, and was playing in first run theatres, a lot of people would see it who would know nothing about MS and just have the old misconceptions confirmed; MS=wheelchair=despair and agony, and add to that – death. I wish they had either done a lot more in the film on the MS or a lot less. I continue to run into the old perception of MS and feel the

MS Society should have put out some kind of disclaimer when the film first came out to correct any misconceptions.

My other big concern, the effect on the newly diagnosed, who may not know how incomplete the picture of MS in the film is. Again, it's not the film's job to inform them, but because this one case will give the wrong impression if generalized, I think the MS Society needed to provide a counter perspective.

Are you worried about the public perception of MS? It's one of the reasons I've done so much writing around the topic, a favourite worry of mine. How do you think we can bring the public image up to date? Please send solution in return mail.

So what public image should we present? There isn't one fits all to be had, unfortunately. The physical symptoms are no less varied than the psychological; both depend at least partially on how long the person in question has had the disease. There are good arguments for taking the cheery approach, the smiling optimist who will not be undone by the disease. But I've also heard compelling arguments for telling it like it is, sharing with people the ugly side. "If we don't tell them, how will they know?"

In the end, we each tell it as we see it; if enough of us are talking, the public will get a composite picture, an understanding of the lack of absolutes or easy generalizations.

Easy to say, but I still have a hard time accepting some points of view, it seems.

Linda to Julie:

Then there's a half page article in the Vancouver Sun (our major city newspaper) by a slightly irrational man with MS who says things like . . . "Imperfect human life, the chronically ill and the disabled, is worth less in Canada than the healthy life," and on and on and on. Again, I thought of that someone, the eavesdropper, as you were saying you hadn't caught the reaction of people with disabilities; this provided perhaps the most outrageous statement of "Poor us, we're the victims here" that I've seen to date, a good one to share with you. Full of rage, I immediately started planning a letter to the editor. But cooled down once I considered the stress on me to keep involved with the topic, of putting myself in the ring, so to speak. "Let it go!" I've learned to do that in the last ten years.

Julie to Linda:

My wish in regard to the public perception is this, that we PwMS are the same people we used to be. That we all have been given a challenge to deal with, and do so in many individual styles, as we are individual people. Though most of what comes with MS is something we would gladly give up, there are a few blessings tucked in as rewards. It takes a long time to be able to recognize them, and then even longer to know what to do with them. I have become so much more sensitive to and appreciative of everyone and everything that is part of my life. Perhaps, because I was always busy, and missed little things that I now have plenty of time to see and experience. I savor every aspect of relationships that were, in the past, important and wonderful, but now, have indescribable dimensions. In the past, I was concerned that my personal contribution to the world should be demonstrated by career accomplishments and educational pursuits, and of course, that my children should learn from parents striving always for goals and to do what is right. My family has always been close and there has always been a lot of love, but I must say, it has been magnified ten fold since MS came to our house. When I hear conversations among people complaining about spouses, children, jobs, aging, and on and on, I immediately think that maybe they aren't seeing the big picture. Perhaps, it's the fact that even simple activities can involve complex planning for PwMS and so we deeply and gratefully regard simplicity, and most of all, we have learned to love it! I don't want anyone feeling sorry for me, BUT, I feel bad that this acquired, expanded purview of life and all of the wonderful things in it, sometimes doesn't fully mature until something like MS slows us down. Then we certainly can look closer at the little stuff.

CONSENSUS

How my e-mail buddies cooperated in my MS education

> *Usually the progression in mobility aids is from cane to walker to scooter or chair. After years using a scooter, I saw the advantage of a walker when I saw Julie with her panoply of mobility aids. Using her walker I was able to look at things in the gift shop, sitting down when my legs gave out. The light went on in my head and I saw how my world would expand if I had a walker. For those places where the cane alone is too demanding, but the scooter is too much. Or the place I want to go, like shops, is not yet easily accessible. I also knew that using the cane too much has had serious consequences in terms of posture and muscles, as did overuse of the scooter. When I got home to BC I had a good look at the walker Flora was using and got one just like it.*

Linda to Flora and Julie:

Hello, to my mentors, I have seen the error of my ways! You two have shown me the way! I am walking once more!

I bought a walker this past week and am already hoofing it down to the park with it, a distance I haven't done on foot for four years or more. I am ecstatic, my legs less so, as they are being asked to rebuild, recover and rediscover why they're attached to my feet.

You two were very instrumental in this. First, I used Julie's walker when I visited her in Stratford and realized I could not have gone to the Festival without it. Plane travel with my scooter seemed pretty much out of the question. Then at home in Vancouver, I visited Flora and test drove her walker, which felt very handy. I had tried walkers before I opted for a scooter, but never found one that felt right. Now, within a six-week period my e-mail buddies had shown me two which worked for me. And that seat was so handy, so close to my bum, so inviting . . . well, I was hooked! I've been able to do less and less walking in the past months and was fretting about it. Now, I will be able to walk comfortably and confidently, seat available when needed and build up the thigh muscles again. I looked at several and opted for one identical to Flora's.

I feel as I did when I got the scooter, that my world has gotten larger. The walker will allow me to do the little errands where putting the scooter on and off the car is impractical, or where handicapped parking is not assured. I have developed a way I can put the walker in the car myself, so the world is once again my oyster, more or less.

Thank you to you both for your sizeable contribution in this.

WALKIN' AND A'ROLLIN LINDA

Julie to Linda:

I'm so-o-o-o happy for you. You will really appreciate the fact that you can now take a purse with you and even carry bags. I use the basket as well as the handles to contain and hang bags from. You sound ecstatic and that's great. Glad to have been part of the team that got you to shop for one. Enjoy it!!

Flora to Linda:

So congrats on the new walker. To coin a phrase, it will be very supportive. Also easy to stow and a lot easier to get into your car. Along with a heavier workload Alan finds the "light" wheelchair hard to get into the car. So I will save it for use with Handidart and their able and experienced staff, not to mention equipment. It will be fun next time we meet. We can have a chat and rest on real chairs just like most folks.

LIFE WITH MS –
SOME CLOSING THOUGHTS

MS has been part of my life for more than a third of it. Reflecting back, thinking about what it has meant involves real mental digging. I know it's meant a great deal, but find it difficult to put it in words. That's just who I am now, Linda with MS.

And it's hard to think of myself without it, somehow. In the past twenty years I have integrated it into my life, a seamless whole again, though attacks had badly fragmented it. Taking my dog for a walk with my scooter now seems very natural, the way others might view using the car to go shopping. But I still do forget and get reminded, once in a while, that MS is more than an accessory to my life. When, for example, I want to dress up a bit to go out, only to later find out I don't feel comfortable, that washroom visits are a nuisance with skirts and slips and poor balance; I end up wishing I'd worn my slacks and runners. And then I wonder, "Am I that disabled, that I resort to wearing no other shoes but runners?" But I'm lucky, I know, that my case of MS is a relatively light one. There are lots whose MS is progressive. I do wonder how they cope.

I've said a lot about MS on these pages. Those of you with the disease won't be surprised that I've perhaps contradicted myself along the way. Others might just find me a hypocrite. It's very hard, I've found, to say anything about life with MS that remains valid for very long. Nothing about having MS is stable or static, including my feeling about it. So what I say may be true at the time but not when the words get printed. MS puts me always in flux, both physically and emotionally. Sometimes my legs are quite steady, sometimes my mind feels sharp, sometimes my bladder is almost normal. Sometimes not.

Given all that, it's hard to maintain a consistent self-image; I feel as if I am many people, depending on the active symptoms at the time. One idea is, however, a constant. I absolutely will not, absolutely refuse to See Myself as a Victim, My Life as Tragic. I bristle at "Poor You", which to me is both an insult and a challenge. "How dare you think that" I want to yell. Which is not to say that I don't at times feel sorry for myself, don't get frightened about the future and frustrated at the present. But accepting life as a tragedy would be admitting defeat; I gain courage for the struggle at the very thought/fear someone might see me that way. The basis of my positive attitude is pride, perhaps.

There's no doubt, it is a struggle. But I haven't yet heard of a human life which isn't, so I don't feel all that different. My struggle has a name, that's all. It's called fatigue, poor balance, neurogenic bladder, vertigo, memory lapses, walking difficulty, TGN, etc. I do believe in the old adage, "What doesn't kill you makes you stronger," that coping skills can develop only when they become needed.

And if I lose track of who I am now at times, what of friends and family? I can be needy and self-centered during an attack, such as my bout with TGN. Most of the time, though, I'm stubbornly independent. If life with MS makes it difficult for me to know myself, I think it must be far worse for those who are not in the driver's seat.

One of my prevailing goals with this disease is to avoid the use of a wheelchair. In my mind, using a scooter isn't in the same category – I don't use it in the apartment at all, and it has really opened up the world to me in my neighborhood. I still use only handrails in the apartment, but there are days when my legs aren't up to the task I ask of them, and I lurch from handrail to chair to chair. But I will keep doing that, including the occasional fall, as long as possible.

Linda L. Ironside

On a bad day I wonder, "When do I see a reward for all this effort?" Feeling sorry for myself is a weakness I do sometimes indulge in. The answer is too obvious – my reward is my continuing ability to walk, to live alone, to do my own shopping, to find quality in life. Another day, I read a story of a mother who lost two children in a home accident, and I am overwhelmed at the thought. That's got to be worse than anything I have to deal with.

It may be that I will, one day, have to adapt to using a wheelchair inside the apartment. I hate the idea of having to make the kinds of changes that would entail, rearranging furniture, etc., but I know if I have to, I will. I know that I hate inconvenience, have very little patience with the physical logistics of life, of tools and space. Maybe that's something MS will teach me yet – patience.

I like to understand – everything (Is that silly?). I also really like a sense of control in my life, at least an awareness of my choices. So when I wake up with, say, more vertigo than I went to bed with, I want to know WHY, and WHAT I should do about it. That can be a problem. MS is not my only descriptor. I am, for starters, a human being, with all the concomitant foibles, moods, and reactions to things around me. I am a premenopausal woman; most of us, men and women, know what unpredictable, unexplainable symptoms that can bring. I am not only middle-aged, but also aging. Though it's very easy to attribute (blame?) just about anything on MS – moodiness, physical weakness, fatigue, passivity, constipation, headache, poor memory, oversleeping, social discomfort – it is also true that many times the same could be due to hormonal imbalance (menopause) or my age or the weather; a low barometric pressure or extreme heat are very hard to take. I'm left not having a clue as to why I'm feeling like I'm feeling, with the result that I'm totally incapable of doing anything about it, EXCEPT work on my attitude.

I'm my own best counsellor, and have very frequent appointments. I know my mental demons, the thinking that can lead me away from the truth. For example, "I'm too tired and don't want to overdo it again," is a common way I try to avoid exercise. Luckily my 'counselor' knows my tricks – I get away with next to nothing! When I feel there's no reason to keep taking the supplements, keep doing the exercises, keep going to TCM appointments, my counselor reminds me something is keeping me going, and that apart from the MS, I have no medical complaints at all. That attitude refresher restores my confidence and strength. And also helps me look at the half full part of my glass, not only the part which is half empty.

"Find calmness!" is another of my counselor's mantras. Things that never used to now make me tense and things which make me tense invite worsening of symptoms – bladder dysfunction, poor balance, and jitteriness. I depend on Valerian, a natural tranquilizer; I also actively try to avoid situations which I know to be stressful, and I always, I mean *always*, without exception, get the sleep or rest I need. My body has taught me I pay too heavily for any excess. Burning the candle at both ends now means less than nine hours sleep in a day or no midday nap. Radical, eh?

I don't hate everything about MS. I have always been happiest when my life had challenge, stimulation and variety. I am easily bored and easily driven. My worst fear is a boring life, one where nothing significant seems to happen. I want a life with intensity. After my horrendous ordeal with TGN (facial pain) was over, I remarked that life suddenly felt a little boring, that I rather appreciated the drama inherent in pain. For me nothing could be worse than boring, stultifying sameness. I like where MS has brought me – the new insight into myself, new outlook on the world, more mature and deeper understanding of life. And a friend says, "But surely there's an easier way to get all that." No, sadly, I don't think so. Maybe for others, but I think I needed a very loud wake-up call, something to really shake me to the core.

People say, "Wouldn't it be wonderful if they found a cure" or "I'm sure there'll be a cure soon." I get tired just thinking about it. I've spent twenty years adapting to my new reality. Learning to live with a multitude of changes. I've left my career stream. I've taken up new interests, such as my writing, have new kinds of relationships. Could I go back and pick up the pieces of where I was twenty years ago? I don't think so. It would not be returning to the old reality, it would perforce be another new reality. Just when I'm getting used to this one. Just when I get all the boxes unpacked and the new place painted and decorated the way I like it, I have to pull up stakes and move again. Oh no!

Putting together a book on MS has, to be honest, really pushed my focusing-on-MS boundary. After a couple of years of writing, another one of editing and organizing, I've just about had it with talking about MS. Dealing with MS is, for me, just a means to an end. The end is a challenging, stimulating life. Learning to cope with MS is the means to having that kind of life, even with physical limitations.

What's next? Luckily, I really don't know. If I did, I might be prone to spending precious time now planning and preparing, making endless lists. People with MS aren't essentially different than others in that regard; no one has the details of their life as a senior or as a very old senior. But those of us with MS have more possibilities penciled in, more possible scenarios to worry about. Fear is a closer companion. But I doubt it could be worse than what I've gone through, group home, depression, etc. to get here, where I am today. I have faith that I will be able to cope, to find some peace and joy.

If life is a journey, MS is a side road I took some time ago which took me in a different direction than I had planned, but which has been, nonetheless, not altogether without interest. Once I was well along the side road, there was nothing for it but to settle in and see what it was all about. I do wonder where the main road would have led me. But it's not as if I've been kicked off the road altogether or fallen in the ditch. I'm on a less well-traveled path, and have no map, but the important thing is I'm still alive, and still traveling. I may not like the destination when I get there, but then the same could be said of those still on the main road. This road is unpaved and very uneven, so I tire more easily than I might have and cover less ground. *But* I am still on a road, meeting people, seeing new things, being stimulated and challenged. My life, even with MS, remains very much one of quality.

Linda L. Ironside

ABOUT THE AUTHOR

Linda Ironside has been a professional educator all of her working life, as a language teacher and consultant. She has an MA from Simon Fraser University in Burnaby, BC, in English as a Second Language, and Educational Administration. Her thesis was on "Chinese and Indo-Canadians in Vancouver – their views on Education."

Her writing career started in BC with professional newsletters. She was first published in Canada when the Vancouver Sun ran a number of articles she wrote while teaching in China; two professional articles also appeared in the Zhongshan (Sun Yat-Sen) University Foreign Language English Journal. Once back home, she wrote human interest articles, such as one on gun control, but gradually focused more on health and disability, including a lengthy report on her experience with acupuncture treatments, which was a 2-page spread in the Vancouver Sun.

Since childhood, she has always been heavily involved in volunteering. One of the contributions she has made to the MS Society in BC is a regular column for the MS Bulletin called "Claude and Friends".

Before taking a disability pension, she was employed as an ESL instructor at Douglas College in New Westminster, BC. She has always enjoyed travel and exposure to other cultures; this led to her teaching in China and consequently being diagnosed there. Her last international trip was to Chile.

Her positive attitude makes this inspiring, uplifting reading for those with MS or any other health-related challenge.

FROM THE PUBLISHER

Linda Ironside's book, *Sharing MS*, is the second in a new series inspired by her and other female authors, that well deserves to be included in the designation, "White Knight's Remarkable Women."

She shares with two other women with MS, and with the reader details of her life as she copes with the daily challenges which MS presents. Life for this professional educator has not unfolded as she would have chosen. But she has always seen MS as a challenge and sought to maintain quality of life in spite of it. From the period of diagnosis in China to her present day volunteerism and freelance writing, she has remained actively engaged in life. The first part of her book is a selection of her personal essays, providing her observations, on life with MS and disability. These perceptions are insightful and uplifting.

The second part of the book brings together the frank e-mail correspondence that occurred with two other women. Like the author, both had successful careers which were stopped short by MS. Their positive attitude makes this inspiring reading for those dealing with MS or any other health-related challenge. The book will be enlightening for those personally affected, their families, friends and acquaintances, as well as those who are are health professionals.

To realize that MS affects more women than men, that it is hereditary, affects people in many different ways, and that it occurs more often in countries as one lives further away from the equator, provides an interesting context for the personal correspondence of these three women in North America (one lives in the US).

Linda L. Ironside

Ironside's book deserves the attention of everyone, especially those who are related to someone with this pernicious disease.

White Knight, Canada's newest publisher of social issue books is proud to bring this new author into the public spotlight.

Bill Belfontaine
Publisher

ADDITIONAL INFORMATION AND RESOURCES

Multiple Sclerosis Society
of Canada
1000 - 250 Bloor Street East
Toronto, Ontario M4W 3P9
416 922-6065

Multiple Sclerosis Society
of USA
1000 - 250 Bloor Street East
Toronto, Ontario M4W 3P9
416 922-6065

Web site: www.mssociety.ca

Toll-free to MS Society division offices
1-800-268-7582

Atlantic Division
71 Isley Avenue, Unit 12
Dartmouth, Nova Scotia B3N 1L5
902 468-8230

Saskatchewan Division
150 Albert Street
Regina, Saskatchewan S4R 2N2
306 522-5600

Quebec Division
1500 - 666 Sherbrooke Street West
Montreal, Quebec H3A 1E7
514 849-7591

Alberta Division
10104 79th Street
Edmonton, Alberta T6A 3G3
780 463-1190

Ontario Division
1000 - 250 Bloor Street East
Toronto, Ontario M4W 3P9
416 922-6065

British Columbia Division
1600 - 1130 West Pender Street
Vancouver, British Columbia
V6E 4A4
604 689-3144

Manitoba Division
400 – 141 Bannatyne Avenue
Winnipeg, Manitoba R3B 0R3
204 943-9595

The Multiple Sclerosis Society of Canada is an independent, voluntary health agency and does not approve, endorse or recommend any specific topic or therapy but provides information to assist individuals in making their own decisions.